Y0-BZE-570

BEGINNER'S
TAI CHI
CHUAN

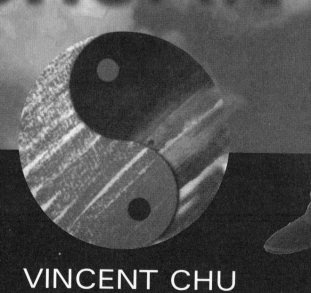

VINCENT CHU

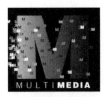

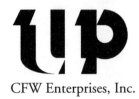

Multi-Media Books

CFW Enterprises, Inc.

DISCLAIMER

Please note that the author and publisher of this book are NOT RESPON-SIBLE in any manner whatsoever for any injury that may result from practicing the techniques and/or following the instructions given within. Since the physical activities described herein may be too strenuous in nature for some readers to engage in safely, it is essential that a physician be consulted prior to training.

First published in 2000 by Multi-Media Books and CFW Enterprises, Inc.

Copyright © 1999 by Vincent Chu

All rights reserved. No part of this publication may be reproduced or utilized in any form or by any means, electronic or mechanical, including photocopying, recording, or by any information storage and retrieval system, without prior written permission from Unique Publications.

Library of Congress Catalog Number: 00-132145
ISBN: 1-892515-17-2
Distributed by:
Unique Publications
4201 Vanowen Place
Burbank, CA 91505
(800) 332–3330

First edition
05 04 03 02 01 00 99 98 97 1 3 5 7 9 10 8 6 4 2
Printed in the United States of America
Design by George Foon
Edited by Mark V. Wiley

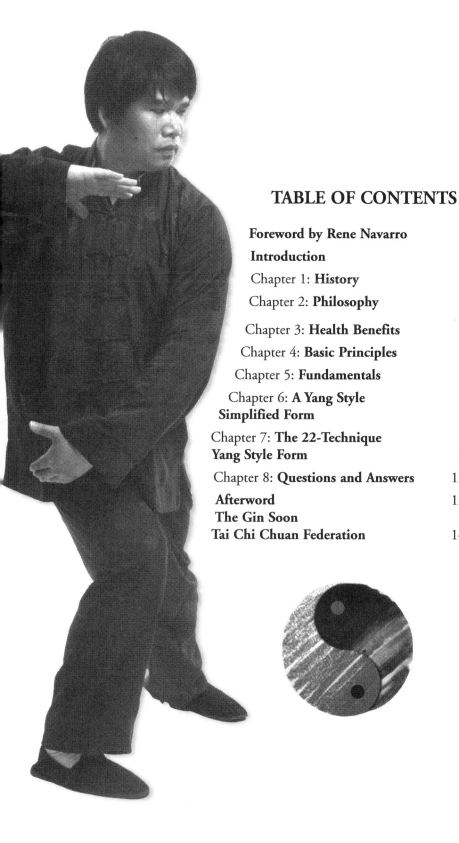

TABLE OF CONTENTS

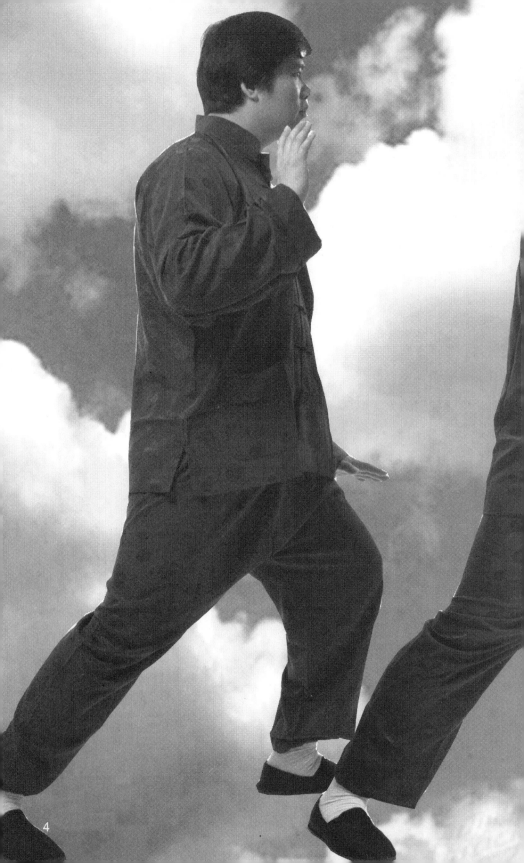

FOREWORD

By Rene J. Navarro, Lic.Ac., Dipl.Ac.

I do not remember meeting Vincent Fong Chu in June of 1986 when I first dropped by the Gin Soon Tai Chi Club. Actually, I do not remember the first time I met him.

Fong, as Vincent is fondly called, is a silent master. An excellent listener, he manages to stay in the background while he observes. Unlike other teachers, who can mount a theatrical production while they are coaching, Fong speaks softly, often conveying his message with a few words. He can rebuke you with a guffaw or with the tilt of an eyebrow.

Fong loves to write his ideas about tai chi chuan and has been published a lot. I had the privilege of editing his many articles. He tantalizes you with the profound, albeit little, information he conveys and irritates you with his self-confidence.

It can be exasperating to interview Fong. I've sat with him for several hours on a few Sunday mornings and when I listened to the tapes, there wasn't much there except my voice and a few inaudible whispers from him. His opinions were brilliant though; unfortunately, the small tape recorder wasn't sensitive enough to record his words.

It is in push hands that Fong articulates his rich knowledge of tai chi chuan. When he pushes, everybody watches. I have seen many masters (both personally and in video tape) and read many books about pushing, but only Fong and his father Gin Soon Chu have the repertoire of push hands techniques that I have only read about in the classics. Fong, who has a facility for English, can also explain what he is doing in terms of the variety of *fa jing* techniques that are mentioned in the tai chi chuan classics. His techniques run the gamut of the 30-odd *fa jing* system, conceivable variations and styles, from the most basic to the most complicated, from the slow to the fast. He can show the most obvious or the most mystical.

I've studied classical Yang family tai chi chuan since late 1989 in the Gin Soon Tai Chi Club. The school is small. Ten to 20 students come usually. It is not rare to see only four or five students. You don't have the SRO classes that are common in other schools, where the master seems to be a director conducting a high-strung theater workshop or a street barker pitching his goods.

Each student is privately coached for 10 to 30 minutes by Chu Sifu or Fong or one of the senior students.

When I began studying tai chi chuan in 1968, in Manila's Chinatown, the students arrived at the club and imitated the form. There wasn't much correction done. Somehow, we were able to memorize the entire form through repetition. It was the same practice in the Luneta Park in Manila and, I noticed, in the other parks in China and the United States.

But at the Gin Soon Tai Chi Club, there is a close attention to the execution of the form. When students finish the solo form, they are subjected to corrections, at least two, of the entire form before they start pushing hands or moving on to any other form in the system.

Much more than any instructor I've seen, Vincent is very particular about alignment and postures. He emphasizes slowness and repetition. Whenever he teaches me, he asks me to repeat the form, not once but many times, until I am ready to drop.

Vincent is quite knowledgeable about tai chi chuan, especially classical Yang family style. He rarely talks, but his knowledge is deep and various. During our private discussions, he would show me certain forms which I thought were lost.

How did the old solo form of the Yang family look? I would ask. He won't answer immediately, but a few days later, he would do a form I haven't seen before.

What is the sword form for? I would ask. It is for fighting somebody who has a weapon, he would say. But nobody carries any weapons around, I would protest. He would say, it helps you extend your *chi,* and then clam up. Hey, what's the secret here? I would mutter.

How do I learn the applications of the solo form? Through push hands and *fa jing,* he says.

He doesn't provide much explanation.

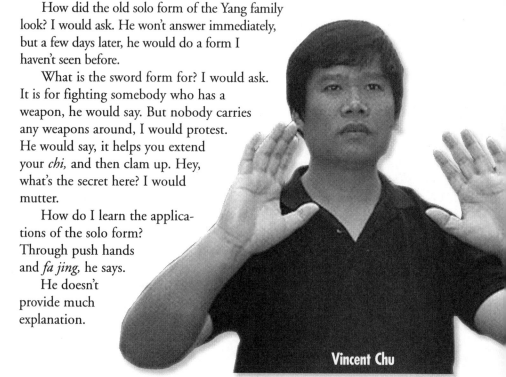

Vincent Chu

His answers come in short, pithy statements. But from my conversations with him, he can go deep into the Classics. His explanations, when they do come, are profound—more profound than any I have seen in writing—and they are backed by a demonstration of the technique.

When he was a child, Vincent Chu began studying the classical tai chi chuan of the Yang family from his father, Master Gin Soon Chu. I would estimate he is now in his late 40s, although he looks at least a decade younger (he won't say exactly how old), so he has been studying tai chi chuan for over at least three decades. Aside from his father and Ip Tai Tak, he has also studied with Grandmaster Yeung (Yang) Sau Chung (the heir and firstborn of Yang Cheng Fu) and several other masters in China.

He trained in the traditional way, through repetition of the forms and techniques. Often, he would stay in one corner and repeat a technique a number of times. Or he would do the left side of a form.

Vincent studied different forms from the old repertoire. At first, I was surprised to see certain forms that I had never seen before. We were alone in the club, working out separately. He would say he was just improvising but later on he would say that he was doing a Yang family form. I should not have been surprised because Vincent belongs to the lineage of the Yang family, trained by his father who was trained by Yeung Sau Chung. He is not your run of the mill teacher, but a real master of the lineage. He isn't your one- or two-form instructor who insists it's going to take the student 20 years to learn what he teaches.

Vincent divides the classical Yang family forms into three segments: 1) Fist forms. Among these are the new solo fist form (which Yeung Cheng Fu choreographed to make tai chi chuan more accessible and easier to learn), push hands, cheung chuan, fast tai chi, 2-man set, 13 animal set, tai chi chuan chi kung, and the old solo fist form; 2) Weapons forms. Included in this category are staff, spear (several forms), knife/broadsword (3 forms), sword (2 forms), and halberd; and 3) Power development forms.

Presented in this book, however, is Vincent's own idea of how a short beginning fist form should be. It's a form he has taught for many years and found important in teaching the fundamental postures of tai chi chuan. Actually, he choreographed this form as a special, and easy-to-remember routine for beginners.

I've seen him do the form many times. Although it contains movements from the solo fist form, it's different from other short forms of tai chi chuan in many ways.

How should it be done?

Let Fong show you.

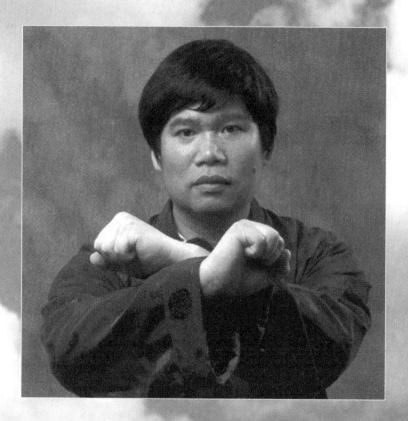

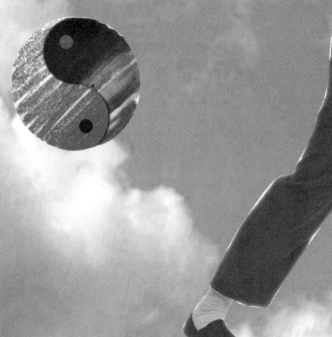

INTRODUCTION

The tai chi chuan routine presented in this book is the result of my teachings at the Brookline Adult and Community Education Program. I began to teach this program in February of 1984. At that time, the program only offered nine-week classes, which makes it impossible to complete the entire solo form of the Yang style. Thus, it was during the first three years teaching in this program that I only taught the first section of the solo form. During this time, many students came to me and complained that they felt there were too many repetitive movements in the form, which made the form difficult to remember.

In an attempt to remedy this, in 1987 I introduced to the class the 24-movement simplified tai chi chuan form that developed in mainland China in 1956. Unfortunately, when it came to the movement "lower the snake body and side kick," many students found it quite difficult to perform. Moreover, I found the 24-movement form to also be too long to learn in a nine-week course.

From these experiences and a number of other reasons, I developed a short tai chi chuan routine that is both easy to remember and long enough for a nine-week class.

In 1988, I began to teach this new short routine based on some of the easy movements of the Yang family style. It turned out to be pretty good. With minor changes, the students find it much easier to learn and remember. Over the next few years, many more students approached me with their video cameras in hand and asked to record my short routine. The requests increased in volume over time and so I decided to do a program that would be made available for many people. In 1991, with the help of Mr. Tom Tetreault, I filmed a tai chi chuan instructional program on Brookline Access Television called "Tai Chi with Vincent Chu." With the help of this program, more people were given access to tai chi chuan in the Greater Boston Area.

It is a result of the classes, the television program, and the many articles I have written for various martial arts magazines that my abbreviated form has reached the eyes and ears of many people. With this exposure came many, many requests to teach the form around the world. While I travel as much as possible, it was felt that publishing an instructional book on the subject would be the best means of promoting the art, thus making it accessible to the many people who are interested in learning it.

Since the English language is a barrier for my father, he spends most of his teaching time on practical issues rather than on tai chi theory. He tells his students that the tai chi chuan theories developed through years of practice. Moreover, a theory developed by one person does not necessary hold true for another person. Therefore, my father encourages each student to develop their own theories from their experiences. He sees himself as a tai chi chuan instructor, not as a communicator or promoter—a job left to his students and myself. Since I posses the direct lineage, the responsibility of carrying the tradition of the Yang style ahead will rest on my shoulders.

This book is divided into six chapters: Chapter One presents the history of Yang style tai chi chuan from its inception to the present day; Chapter Two presents the philosophical underpinnings of tai chi chuan; Chapter Three offers an overview of the many and vast health benefits gained from the practice of this movement discipline; Chapter Four offers an overview of the basic principles of tai chi chuan and how they relate to the movements; Chapter Five presents the fundamentals of the system, from how to stand and breath to how to move and think; Chapter Six puts it all together by illustrating and discussing the short form of Yang style that I have constructed; and Chapter Seven offers the most frequently asked questions that have been posed regarding tai chi chuan and my answers to them. The book then concludes with some final thought.

I would like to thank my father, who taught me this wonderful art of tai chi chuan. Without his kindness and encouragement as a father, and patience, demands, and discipline as a teacher, I would not have been able to do it.

I appreciate Ms. Linda Larson and Mr. Irving Schwartz, director of Brookline Adult, Community, and Education Program, for helping me to improve myself. And also the staff as EIKOS, who opened their arms to embrace any question and problem I had as an inexperienced teacher in tai chi chuan.

Finally, this book could not have be completed without the contribution of my friends and students, David Gabbe and Tony Zhu.

Thank you all!

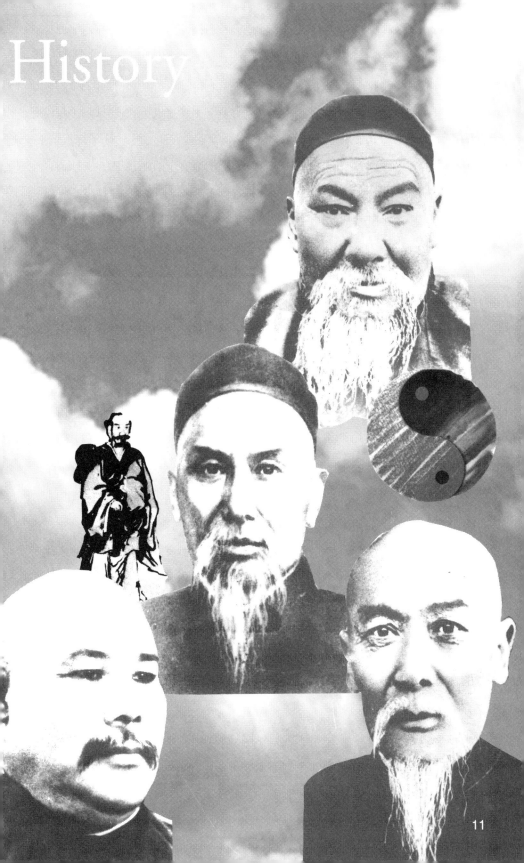

History

11

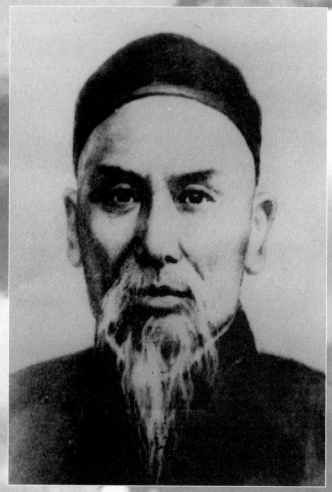

Yang Lu Chan

Chapter 1

HISTORY

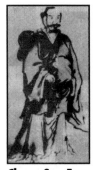

Chang San Feng

There are many stories in terms of who created tai chi chuan. Commonly, it is said that the creator was a Taoist priest name Chang San Feng. He was said to have been a master of Shaolin kung-fu who later combined the art with the philosophy of Taoism, creating a style that does not rely on physical strength, but mental concentration and internal energy. Today, this new style is known as tai chi chuan.

Long before Chang San Feng, there were exercises practiced among various Taoist priests during the Tang dynasty (A.D. 618–905). Hsa Suan-Ping, a native of An-Huei province in southeast China, practiced an exercise called *san hsi chi* (37 movements exercise); Li Tao Tze practiced an exercise called *hsien-tien chuan* (the stage before the universe was created); in the Liang dynasty (A.D. 907–921), Hen Kon Yu practiced an exercise called nine little heavens; and Hu Chin-Tze (n.d.) practiced an exercise called *hu tien fa* (the stage after the universe was created). Chang San Feng is credited as the creator of tai chi chuan because he was the one who spread the art to help all people enjoy a longer and healthier life. From martial art techniques he developed a body, mind, and spirit discipline.

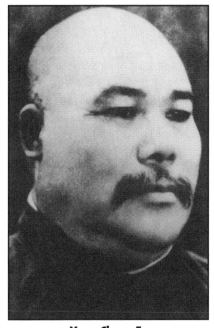

Yang Cheng Fu

After Chang San Feng, this internal discipline exercise was passed on among the Taoist society for many generations. In the 16th century, Wang Tsung Yueh was famous for his skill in tai chi chuan. Wang in turn passed his skill to his student Chiang Fah (1574–?). Chiang had two students who carried on the skills, of which Chen Chang Hsin (1771–1853) was the successor of the art. Chen passed his skill on to his student Yang Lu Chan (1799–1872). Yang popularized tai chi chuan in Beijing and then passed his skill on to his two sons, Yang Pan Hou (1837–92) and Yang Chien Hou (1839–1917). Yang Chien Hou passed his skill on to his two sons, Yang Shao Hou (1862–1930) and Yang Cheng Fu (1883–1936). It was as a result of Yang Cheng Fu's teaching that tai chi chuan

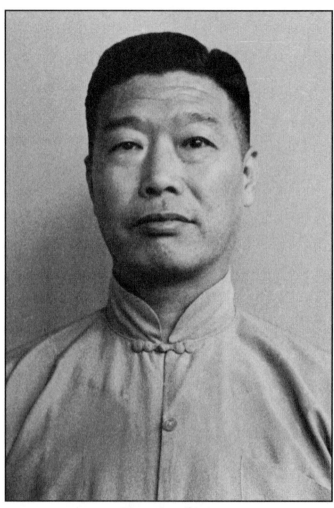

Yeung Sau Chung

became popular, not just in North China but all around the country. Yang Cheng Fu passed his skill on to his eldest son, Yeung Sau Chung (1910–85).

After the Communist party took over China in 1949, many well-known tai chi chuan masters moved from China to Hong Kong, Taiwan, and Singapore. My father's teacher, Mr. Yeung (Yang) Sau Chung, was the eldest of four sons of the late Yang (Yeung) Cheng Fu. When Cheng Fu died in 1936, Sau Chung was 26 years old and his three brothers were 15, 10, and eight, respectively. Although Cheng Fu's three younger sons live and are active in teaching the family style of tai chi chuan today, Sau Chung was the only son to truly carry the tradition and transmission from their father.

After Yeung Sau Chung settled down on Hong Kong Island, he had three daughters in his second marriage, and accepted Mr. Ip Tai Tak as his first disciple among thousands of students.

In 1956, to improve his health, my father, Gin Soon Chu, started learning tai chi chuan under master Lai Hok Soon, who was the student of Yeung Cheng Fu and Yeung Sau Chung. I met one of my father's former roommates, Mr. Kwan Chop, one day in October of 1987. He said that he was one of six people living with my father in the early '50s in a small apartment in Kowloon,

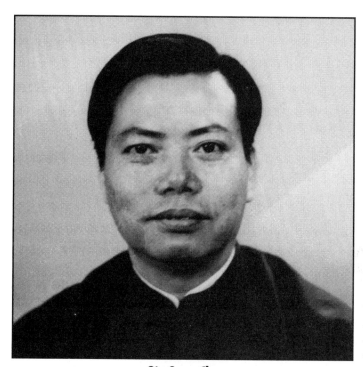

Gin Soon Chu

Hong Kong. The building had no elevator; everyone who lived in that building had to take the stairs and my father was always the last one to reach their apartment on the fifth floor. Mr. Kwan said that my father's health was so poor that he had to stop and rest on every floor. It was later that my father said that if not for tai chi chuan, he would not be around today.

It was upon the passing of Master Lai in 1964 that my father inherited Master Lai's school. However, in his desire for more advanced training, my father turned the school over to his classmate, Mr. Chan Ping Tim, and became a student of the famous Mr. Yeung Sau Chung, the fourth descendent of the Yang (Yeung) style of tai chi chuan.

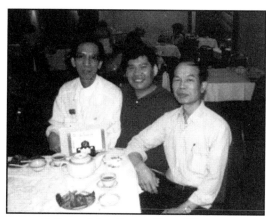

Left to right, Kwan Chop, Vincent Chu and Chan Ping Tim in 1995.

In 1968, my aunt requested that my father come to the United States to helped her manage the Song Hee Restaurant in Boston, Massachusetts. Many people in the Chinese community in Boston knew that my father had been practicing tai chi chuan and encouraged him to teach the art within the community. With the permission of Mr. Yeung, the Gin Soon Tai Chi Club was established in 1969 to promoted Yang style tai chi chuan among Boston's Chinese community.

Since my father came to the United States, he has returned many times to Hong Kong to continue his tai chi chuan training with Mr. Yeung. Finally, in 1977, my father was accepted by Mr. Yeung as his second disciple and given responsibility for the sustenance and propagation of the Yang family style of tai chi chuan in North America.

After the closing of the Song Hee Restaurant in 1976, my father devoted full time to his teaching of tai chi chuan. It was at this time that he began to accept American students, as well as Chinese, as long as they were interested in the art. Although most of the student body at the Gin Soon Tai Chi Club today come from the Greater Boston Area, there are students who come weekly from Rhode Island, New York State, Connecticut, and New Hampshire. In addition, international students come to train at the club annually from such places as France, England, Germany, and Italy.

I was introduced to the wonderful art of tai chi chuan as a very young child. I spent a lot of time practicing before and after school. My father told me that I had to learn it so that I could later teach my brothers. When my father taught me, he wanted me to repeatedly practice the same movement over-and-over many times before I moved on to a new one. It is as a result of this hard training that now when a student comes to me and says his leg hurts, I know exactly which muscle is affected by which stance. When a student tells me he has black-and-blue skin as a result of pushing too hard, I know exactly how many days it will take for the discolored mark to disappear.

"It was later that my father said that if not for tai chi chuan, he would not be around today."

By the time I reached the age of 16, I had already learned the solo form, various push hand exercises, the knife form, and the sword form, and became an assistant in my father's school. Throughout the years, I have taught many students at my father's school here in Boston's Chinatown.

By the early 1980s, I had published several articles on tai chi chuan in *Tai Chi* and *Inside Kung-Fu* magazines.

In 1984, I was invited to Vancouver, Canada to conduct a workshop on tai chi chuan. It was the first time that I conducted such a class by myself and I enjoyed it very much. I enjoyed the teaching experience so much that as soon as I returned to Boston I approached the Brookline Adult and Community Education Program to offer them my services as a tai chi teacher. Over the past 12 years, I have had the great opportunity to offer tai chi chuan workshops in the United States and aboard.

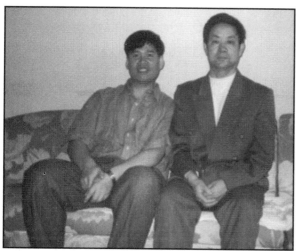

Vincent with Tang Shan Fu in China.

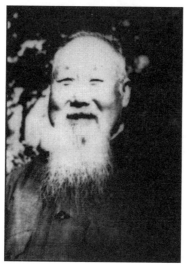

Tsau Li Shu

Although Yang style tai chi chuan is the most popular of the five tai chi styles in the world today, there are relatively few masters of the art openly teaching it. And so, to improve and advance my knowledge of Yang style tai chi chuan, in September of 1984 my father sent me to Hong Kong to learn from his teachers, Grandmaster Yeung Sau Chung. In 1992, I met Mr. Ip Tai Tak in Hong Kong and Mr. Tang Shan Fu in Tai Yuen, China. Mr. Tang introduced me to his teacher, Professor Fang Ning, who learned his tai chi chuan from Tsau Li Shu. Tsau was one of the senior students of Yang Cheng Fu, and Tsau was famous for his tai chi chuan skill in Beijing area.

PHILOSOPHY

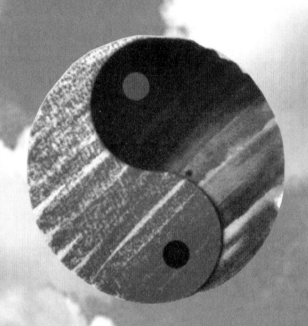

Chapter 2

PHILOSOPHY

Tai chi chuan literally translates as the "grand ultimate boxing." It is called this based on the philosophy of tai chi. The term "tai chi" first appeared in the *I Ching* or *Book of Changes,* which was published more than two-thousand years ago. In this book, it is said that tai chi came form *wu chi* or the stage of nothingness. While in motion, the *wu chi* created tai chi and became the mother of *yin* and *yang.*

It is very common nowadays to see a tai chi chuan symbol in many kinds of print media. To familiarize yourself with the symbol, here is what it looks like: a circle divided into two equal fish-like components. One half of the component is white and is called *yang,* and the other half of the component is black and is called *yin.* Within the white, there is the black dot. Within the black, there is the white dot. The *yin* component represents anything in the universe that is female, passive, negative, night, left, bottom, or soft. The *yang* component represents the direct opposite, such as male, active, positive, day, right, top, or hard. Therefore, *yin* and *yang* are not only a pair of opposites but complementary forces in the universe. In essence, the symbol has four distinguished properties. They are:

1. Opposite: One can see from the symbol that the two components are directly opposite one another in every way.

2. Complementary: One can see from the symbol that these two components complement each others. One can't exist without the other. For example, one can not distinguished a right hand without recognizing that there is a left hand. There is no day without night. There can be no reference to what is female without the existence of something male.

3. Balance: Another look at the symbol reveals that the circle is divided by a serpentine line and two opposite dots. This explains that nothing is absolute and nothing is pure. As indicated in this symbol, the *yin* component possess properties of the *yang* component, and the *yang* component possesses properties of the *yin* component.

Let us take a look at the concept of balance in reference to our lives. Let's take 12 months for example. We know that the Summer is hot and the Winter is cold. We do not go directly from Summer into Winter or Winter into Summer. Rather, we have the Spring and Fall in between the Summer and Winter.

4. Interaction: This last concept needs a little more imagination to understand. The existence of the serpentine line suggests that the symbol can be interpreted as being in motion. When the two components are in motion, the *yin* component will become the *yang* component and the *yang* component will become the *yin* component. We see this happening all of the time in politics, business, among friends, among family members, and among party members.

From this concept of struggle, everything evolves. This is what the Taoists call from one to two, two to four, four to eight, and eight to ten-thousand, or from *wu chi* to tai chi, from tai chi to the four phenomenon, from the four phenomenon to the *pa kua,* and from the *pa kua* to ten-thousand things.

Since tai chi chuan was created by a Taoist priest, one can see why some people insist that the art is the fruit of Taoism. The major text on Taoism, the *Tao Te Ching,* was written by Lao Tzu, who lived around the fourth century B.C. Lao said that all things evolved from the Tao and to follow the Tao is to act natural according to the laws of the Universe, rather than the artificial.

After one practices tai chi chuan for sometime, they will discover for themselves just how this art utilizes the philosophy of *yin/yang* and how Lau Tzu's concepts of Tao apply to the tai chi chuan movements.

Recently, tai chi chuan theorists have added the concepts of the *I Ching's* hexagrams and the five elements to tai chi chuan, and how they correspond to each of the art's movements.

> **"Since tai chi chuan was created by a Taoist priest, one can see why some people insist that the art is the fruit of Taoism."**

Traditionally, *I Ching* is better known as a group of eight broken and unbroken lines or hexagrams, used to understand the mystery of nature. In tai chi chuan, it is used to represent the eight fundamental directions and energy of movements. The eight major techniques or gates in tai chi chuan are "ward off," "roll back," "press," "push," "pull down," "split," "elbow strike," and "shoulder strike." Tai chi chuan utilizes the five elements (metal, wood, water, fire, and earth) to represent five steeping movement and directions. Taken together, these 13 elements are formally known as 13 postures, and are the foundation upon which all tai chi chuan movements are based and built.

HEALTH
BENEFITS

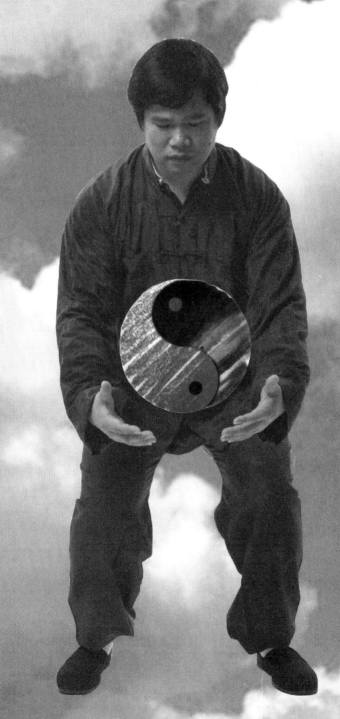

Chapter 3

HEALTH BENEFITS

At dawn each morning, people come together in the Chung Shi Peoples' Park in China to practice tai chi chuan. While I was there, I found three organized groups practicing tai chi chuan, among numerous other forms of physical discipline. Of the three groups of tai chi chuan, I was following the smallest group, in which the members were practicing the 88 movements of the Yang style, also known as the Yang style long form. Many of these tai chi chuan practitioners can explain to you different and yet similar stories as to why and how they started to practice tai chi chuan.

A Mrs. Zhang Shu Lai said that she started practicing tai chi chuan when she was in a rehabilitative hospital. It all began when she was in a car accident, after which it took her many months to recover. During this time, a doctor prescribed the practice of tai chi chuan as her medicine. After a period of practice, she found a speedy recovery. Mrs. Zhang credits tai chi chuan as the reason she is able to walk again. Therefore, she has practiced tai chi chuan religiously every morning for the last three years.

Mr. Lu Chung Fa said that he began practicing tai chi chuan because he was so sick and had such problem with breathing that his doctor recommended he should do some physical exercise in addition to taking his regular medicine. This was 14 years ago, and, as it now turns out, he is the leader of this group practice.

These are but two of the many stories I heard when I was practicing my tai chi chuan with the Chung Shi People's Park Tai Chi Chuan Group in April of 1993 in Canton, China.

Tai chi chuan developed originally as a form of physical health discipline by the Taoist society. Many skillful tai chi chuan practitioners were known to have lived well into their old age by simply practicing tai chi chuan. As a direct result of its slow, gentle, and soft movements, a tai chi chuan practitioner can reap many physical benefits, such as better digestion, improved blood circulation, and an increased amount of oxygen intake to aid the body's natural functions. And because of its characteristics, any individual can learn this profound exercise. whether they be a muscular man or slender woman, an active teen or a white-haired senior citizen.

> **"Many skillful tai chi chuan practitioners were known to have lived well into their old age by simply practicing tai chi chuan."**

The mental benefits of practicing tai chi chuan are found in the art's characteristic slowness and softness. A slow and soft movement enables someone to better control their physical movements and relax their body at the same time so that it will reduce the stress and tension cultivated from our hectic, everyday problems.

Medical studies have found that slow, gentle, and soft tai chi chuan movement is good for promoting better blood circulation and has calming effects on the mind. Such movements soften the blood vessels to avoid hardening of the arteries so that it can provide more blood to the organs without additional demands from the heart. The large amounts of oxygen gained from prolonged practice will help one to clear the mind and reduce stress and tension.

It is no wonder why the medical experts in China introduce and encourage people to practice tai chi chuan, an exercise that prepares us to face everyday problems. This is why millions of people practice tai chi chuan and it is still growing strong.

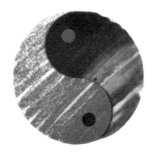

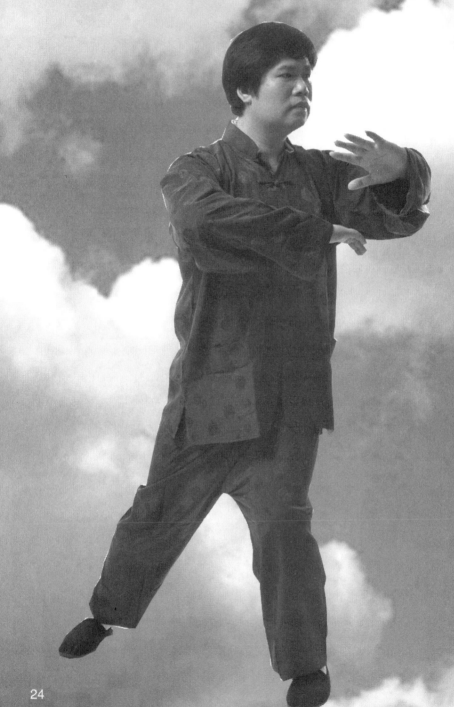

BASIC
PRINCIPLES

Chapter 4

BASIC PRINCIPLES

Yang style tai chi chuan's basic characteristics of movement are natural, relaxed, soft, and open. When one practices tai chi chuan, they feel comfortable, stretched, relaxed, and most importantly, that their body is energetic as the result of better blood circulation. When one observes tai chi chuan practice, they witness a performance of controlled precision, slow and even with grace.

To learn tai chi chuan movement is easy; to master the art of tai chi chuan is difficult. The tai chi chuan classics confirm this difficulty and recommend that a prospective student should obtain oral instruction from a teacher. This means that the instruction should consist of explanation of the principles and demonstration of the movements in relationship to the principles by the teacher.

TO BE SOFT AND RELAXED

The entire body must always be relaxed and soft throughout every movement of the tai chi chuan form. One especially should pay attention to all of the major joints in the body, and keep in mind that relaxation does not mean collapsing the body. Therefore, the body should be supple and without tension in all movements. Relaxation for all movements begins physically as well as mentally.

TO BE SLOW

All tai chi chuan movements should be done slowly so that greater coordination can be possible. When one moves slowly, one can better control muscle movements without harm. When one moves slowly, one tends to pay greater attention to each movement, rather than rushing through them. When one moves slowly, one is better able to appropriately coordinate the breath with the movements. When one moves slowly, one will improve his patience. Therefore, slowness develops exactness.

TO BE NATURAL AND SPONTANEOUS

Tai chi chuan is an outgrowth of Taoism—the study of life and nature. In order for this art to follow Taoism, then, one must practice tai chi chuan naturally and spontaneous. In this case, "naturally" means that one should hold the head upright, the back straight, the arms naturally at their sides, with all the joints moving loosely together without tightness. If the joints are tight or stiff, inhibited movements will result, thus leading to "slack and jerk." According to Taoism, this means death. Therefore, to be natural and spontaneous mean life.

TO HAVE CONCENTRATION

One should not practice tai chi chuan absentmindedly. Full attention must be given to each and every movement. When you move the right hand, attention should be on that right hand movement.

TO BE COORDINATED

When one is able to coordinate the upper and lower body in movement, one is moving the body as a whole. When this occurs, all of the muscle groups will move together in one motion. When one is moving the body as "one unit," each movement will contain maximum strength and stability.

TO MAINTAIN BALANCE

To maintain balance in movement, one must begin with an understanding of *yin* and *yang*. In this case, *yin* refers to the foot that does not carry the body weight, while *yang* refers to the foot that carries the body weight. When you want to move the left foot, you should shift all of your body weight onto the right foot, and vice-versa.

To maintain balance of inner energy, one must harmonize the hands with the feet, the hip joints with the shoulder joints, and the elbow joints with the knee joints.

To maintain balance in tai chi chuan training, one must practice the tai chi chuan solo form and the tai chi chuan push hands exercises.

To maintain balance mentally, one must execute all of the movements according to these basic principles.

TO BE BOTH EMPTY AND FULL

To be both empty and full means to simultaneously be *yin* and *yang*. The tai chi chuan classics state that one can only fully master the art of tai chi chuan when one truly understands the concept of *yin* and *yang*. This means that while there are only two divisions of things existing in this universal at all times, they embrace many ideas: the two components oppose and yet attach to each other, and one can not exist without the other; the two components are always in a struggle to overcome the other; the two components are constantly seeking out a balance position as there is no clear-cut separation of the components; and the two components constantly exchange position, *yang* becoming *yin* and *yin* becoming *yang*.

TO BE ROOTED AND SUNK

To understand balance, one should begin by first understanding relaxation, then go a step further toward understanding sinking. Sinking is achieved by first dropping one's center of gravity and then lowering the inner energy *(chi)* to the lower abdomen *(tan tien)*. By lowering the center of gravity, one is able to relax the body and all of its joints. Sinking provides better balance. Relaxation provides better sinking.

As one can see from these basic principles, in order for a tai chi chuan practitioner to practice correctly, he/she must begin to understand these basic principles, noting that they are in fact all intimately related to one another.

In sum: nature provides better relaxation; relaxation provides better sinking; sinking provides better balance; balance provides better coordination; coordination provides better empty and full; empty and full provide better slowness; and slowness provides better naturalness.

Chapter 5

FUNDAMENTALS

In order to practice tai chi chuan correctly, a beginner must pay meticulous attention to the body. Following are brief descriptions of each of the major body parts and how they must be held. Following this are brief descriptions of the basic stances and how they must be held.

Body Parts

The head

The head should be keep upright at all times, as if an energy is supporting it. One should not lean the head in any direction. Indeed, when the head is held straight and upright, one is better able to concentrate and focus. This is why the classics state that the head should be held as if "suspend from above."

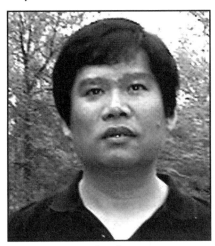

Correct head position

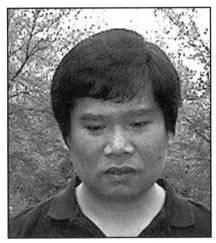

Incorrect head position

The eyes

The eyes are the window that separates the body from its environment. The eyes should be relaxed and look forward and far, thus being able to support the suspension of the head from above. When the mind directs the head to move in a certain direction, the eyes should move there first, the head and body following in turn.

The mouth

The lips should be closed with the tip of the tongue touching the roof of the mouth. This connection will keep the mouth moist, and breathing should be done through the nose slowly and evenly.

The neck

The neck has to be erect so that the head can be upright and the spirit can reach the top of the head. The neck must be relaxed and loose enough so that it can easily turn from side to side without tension.

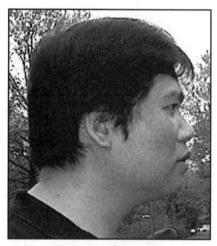

Correct neck position

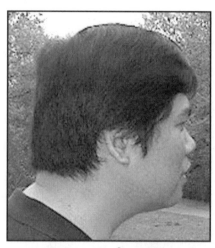

Incorrect neck position

The shoulders

The shoulders are among the major joints of the body. In order to keep the body relaxed at all times, the shoulders should be relaxed and soft, thus keeping the joints loose from lack of tension and the connective tissue agile and elongated. Thus, the shoulders must be kept sunken, relaxed, and agile.

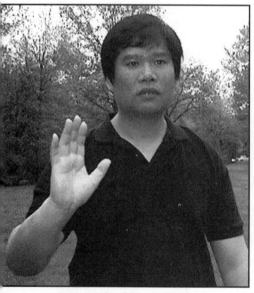

Correct shoulder position

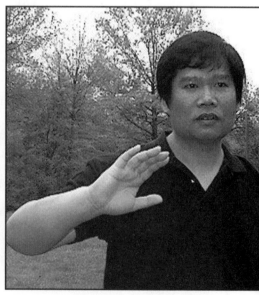

Incorrect shoulder position

The elbows

The elbows are one of the joints that affect the quality of the inner energy *(chi)* movement into the hands. By lowering the elbows, this inner energy can travel more efficient into the hands.

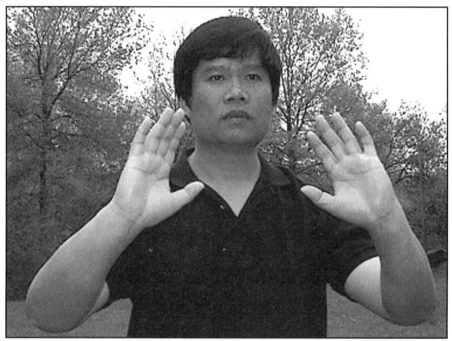

Correct elbow position

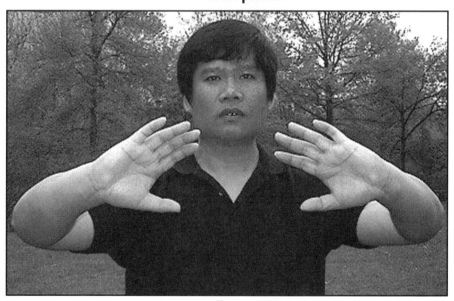

Incorrect elbow position

The hands

In tai chi chuan practices, most of the defensive movements utilize the palm strike. In the Yang family style, the palm is called the "lotus palm" as the five fingers are held open resembling a lotus leaf, and the wrist is bent so that the center of the palm looks outward. Although the fist is not commonly used, it should be loosely clinched together so that it will not inhibit the flow of the inner energy.

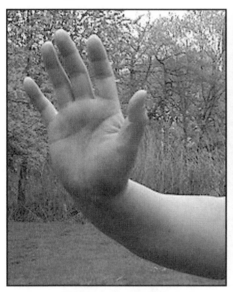

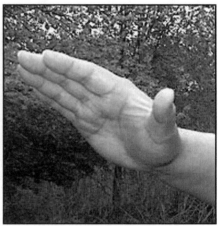

Incorrect palm position

Correct palm position

The fingers

The fingers should be loosely stretched outward and not stuck together.

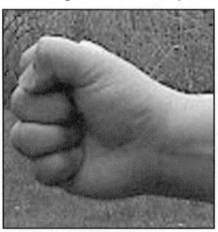

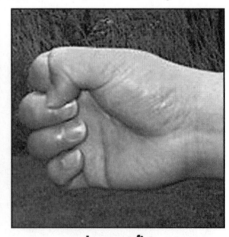

Correct fist

Incorrect fist

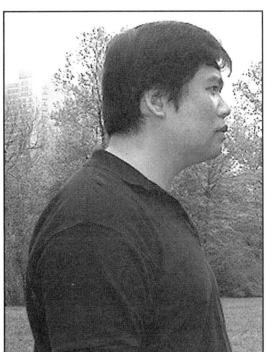

Correct chest and back position

The chest

The chest must be hollow, reducing any tension they may otherwise develop during tai chi chuan practice. When the chest is hollow and tension reduced, the breath is natural and the inner energy is better able sink to the bottom.

The back

The back should be raised in accordance with the hollowing of the chest. In fact, when you raise the back, the chest will automatically hollow. When the back is raised, the inner energy will be stored there and later issued into the hands and fingers.

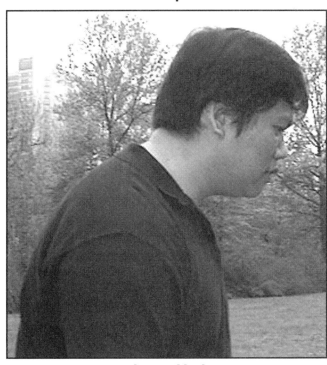

Incorrect chest and back position

The waist

The hips are among the most important joints in the body. Every tai chi chuan movement should begin with the rotation of the waist, which is why the classics call it the "commander." The waist must be loose so that inner energy can easily sink and so that the body can rotate more easily.

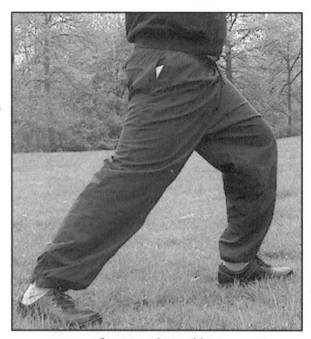

Correct waist position

The buttocks

In order to keep this inner energy sunken, the buttocks must be tucked under so that the tail bone will become straight.

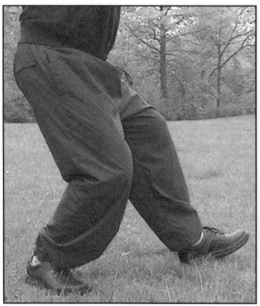

Correct buttock position

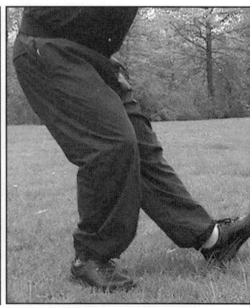

Incorrect buttock position

The groin

In order to keep the inner energy sunken, the groin must be loose and round. When I say round, I am referring to the groin looking more like a U-shape rather than a V-shape.

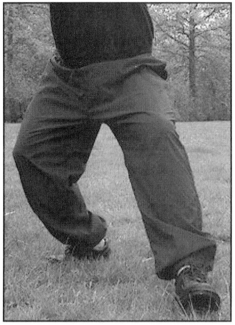

Correct groin position

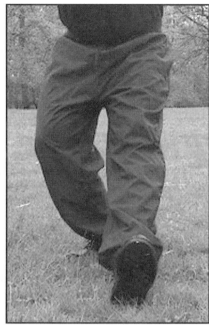

Incorrect groin position

The knees

When you assume any stance, the knees should always be held in line with the toes. Since the knees are a very delicate joint that can be injured quite easily, they should not be twisted.

The feet

In order for the inner energy *(chi)* to exchange with its environment through the bubbling well point *(tan tien)*, the toes must strongly grip the ground. It can help the inner energy sink and provide rootedness in any posture.

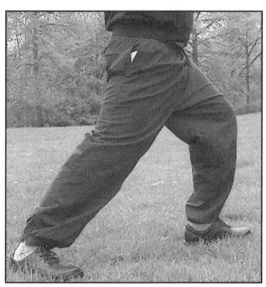

Correct knees position

Stances

All the stances in the tai chi chuan solo form are called *yin/yang* stances. This means that only one foot is needed to support the whole body weight. The foot that is supporting the body weight is called the *yang* foot and the empty-weighted foot is called the *yin* foot. Here are descriptions of some of the stance in the tai chi chuan form.

Forward bow stance

In the forward bow stance, the knee of the front foot is bent to support 60 percent of the body weight. The rear foot is held straight and supports 40 percent of the body weight. Generally speaking, when one assumes this position, one should keep the "three heads" in a straight line (i.e., head, knee, toe). The body should form an inclined posture, as opposed to an upward or leaning posture as seen in many hard-style martial arts. The distance between the feet depends on the length of one's foot and the width between them depends on the width of one's shoulders.

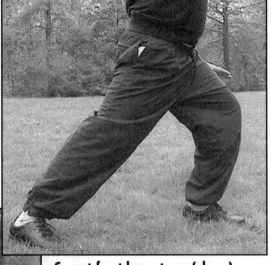

When the left foot is in front, the stance is called the left bow stance. When the right foot is in front, the stance is called the right bow stance. This stance is very common in the tai chi chuan solo form.

Incorrect front bow stance (below)

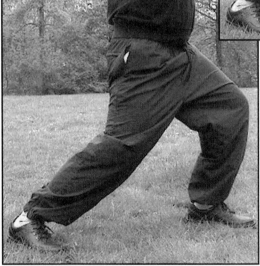

Correct front bow stance (above)

Rear bow stance

In the rear bow stance, 60 percent of the body weight is supported by the rear foot, with the rear knee kept bent. The front foot is held straight, with 40 percent of the body weight resting on it.

What is important in this stance is that the waist be held backward, sinking the weight into the supporting leg. When the weight is supported by the right foot, it is called the right rear bow stance. When the weight is supported by the left foot, it is called the left rear bow stance.

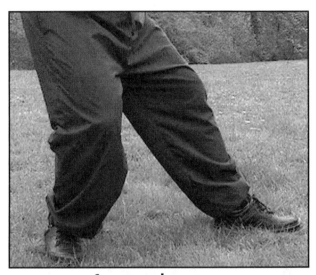

Correct rear bow stance

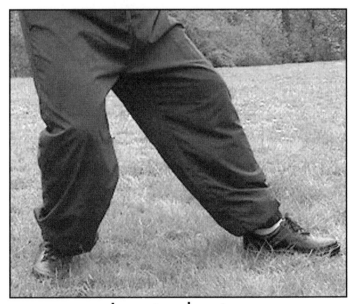

Incorrect rear bow stance

Cat stance

This stance is similar to the rear bow stance except that the toes of the front foot are held off the ground. Whenever one makes a step, it always begins in this stance because of it's agility. As such, it is easier to retreat or plant the whole foot down afterward.

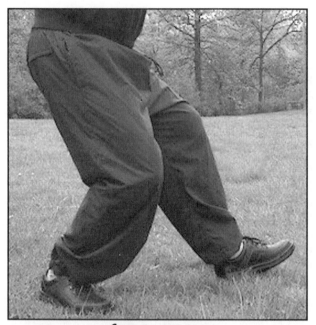

Correct cat stance

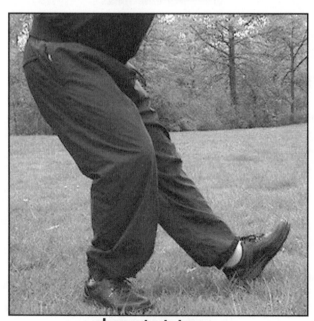

Incorrect cat stance

Rise the horse stance

This stance is similar to the rear bow stance, except that the toes of the font leg touch the ground and most of the body weight is supported by the rear leg. If one trains this stance well, all of their kicking movements will be stable and balanced.

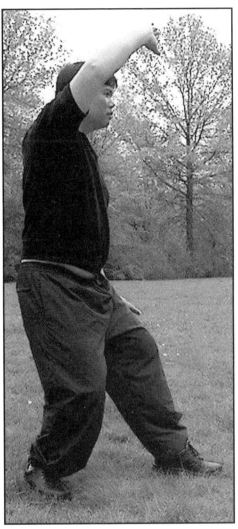

Correct rising horse stance

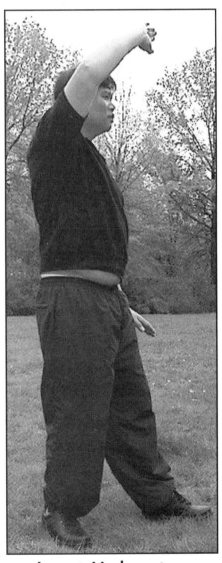

Incorrect rising horse stance

Chapter 6

A YANG STYLE SIMPLIFIED FORM

This 22-movement abbreviated tai chi chuan form is the result of many years of my students' recommendations. Although the form is abbreviated, the essential characteristics found in the Yang style long form, such as open, circulate, comfortable, even, slow, and high stance are also found here.

In developing this form, I removed all of the difficult and kicking movements of the traditional solo form as taught in my father's school, Gin Soon Tai Chi Chuan Federation, so that this abbreviated form is easier for beginning students to remember and practice. However, this form in no way is intended to be a substitute for the traditional Yang family form. This form mainly functions as a stepping stone to tai chi chuan's many profound training methods.

Before going into the description of the form and its 22 movements, I list them all below as a quick reference to them.

NAMES OF THE MOVEMENTS

1. Beginning Tai Chi Chuan
2. Wild Horse Ruffling Its Mane (right)
3. Wild Horse Ruffling Its Mane (left)
4. White Crane Spreads Its Wings
5. Brush Knee and Twist Step (right)
6. Brush Knee and Twist Step (left)
7. Brush Knee and Twist Step (right)
8. Fist Under Elbow
9. Step Backward and Drive Away Monkey (right)
10. Step Backward and Drive Away Monkey (left)
11. Step Backward and Drive Away Monkey (right)
12. Step Backward and Drive Away Monkey (left)
13. Grasp Sparrow's Tail (left)
14. Grasp Sparrow's Tail (right)
15. Left Warding Off
16. Waving Hands like Clouds (3 times)
17. Fair Lady Works on Shuttles (right)
18. Turn Around and Chop
19. Step Forward and Punch
20. Wild Horse Ruffling It's Mane (left)
21. Grasp Sparrow's Tail (right)
22. Closing Tai Chi Chuan

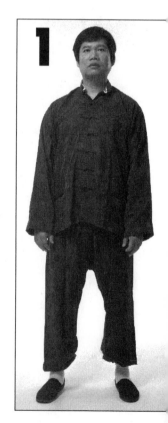

Following is a breakdown and description of each of the 22 movements as they are practiced and performed in this form.

BREAKDOWN OF THE MOVEMENTS
1. Beginning Tai Chi Chuan

A. Begin the form facing south, with both feet pointing forward and held firmly to the ground a shoulders-width apart. The knees are held together loosely. The hands are held relaxed down along the sides of their respective legs *(fig. 1)*.

B. Slowly raise both hands to shoulder level with the palms facing each other *(fig. 2)*.

C. Turn the palms to face down and slowly drop the hands down to each side of the legs with the palms facing downward and the fingers facing forward *(fig. 3)*.

D. Slowly raise your right hand to the right side with its palm facing away from the body. Then raise your left hand up to the chest with its palm facing downward *(fig. 4)*.

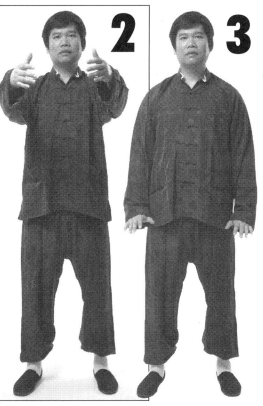

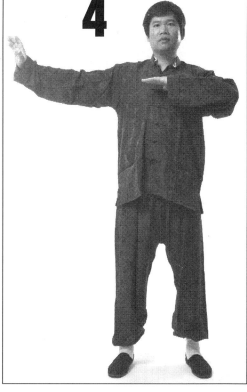

2. Wild Horse Ruffling Its Mane (right)

A. Turn your left foot out and lower your body.

B. Turn your right palm to face upward and move it to your left side until it is under your left hand. *(fig. 5)*

C. Step 45 degrees to the right corner with your right foot. Slowly shift your body weight onto your right foot, while at the same time separating your hands by moving your right hand up and your left hand down *(fig. 6)*.

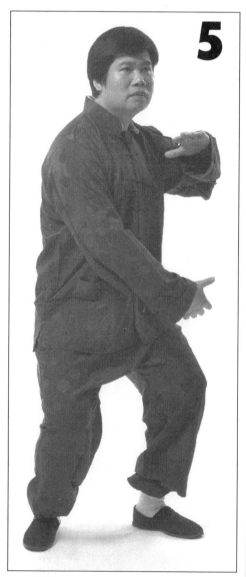
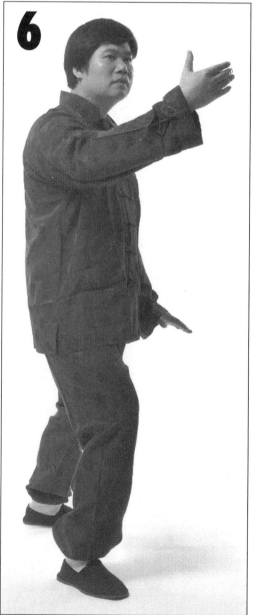

3. Wild Horse Ruffling Its Mane (left)

A. Turn your left palm to face up and move it to the right knee until it is under your right hand. Turn your right hand until its palm faces down *(fig. 7)*.

B. Turn your right foot out and step 45 degrees to the left corner with your left foot. From here, slowly shift your body weight onto your left foot, while at the same time separating your hands so that your left hand moves up and your right hand moves down *(fig. 8)*.

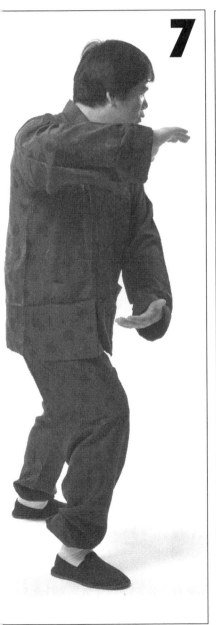 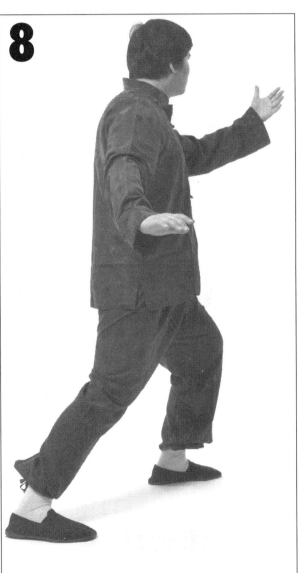

4. White Crane Spreads Its Wings

A. Take a half step with your right foot toward your left foot *(fig. 9)*.

B. Raise your right hand up until it is above your forehead with the thumb pointing down and move your left hand down, with its fingers pointing forward, until it is next to your left leg, *(fig. 10)*.

C. Place your body weight onto your right foot while stepping with your left foot, resting on its toes *(fig. 11)*.

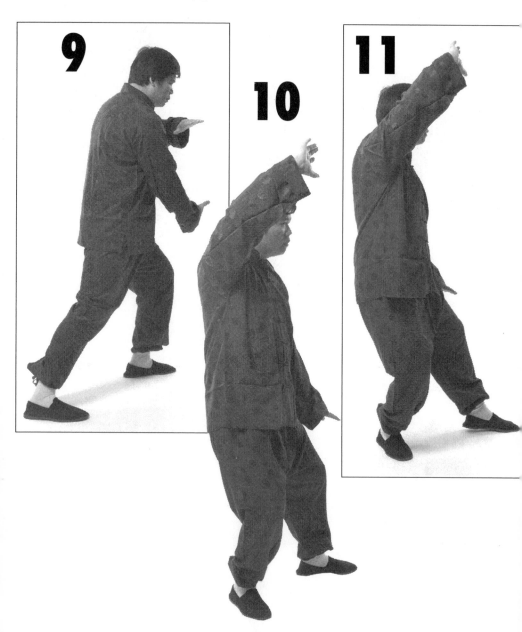

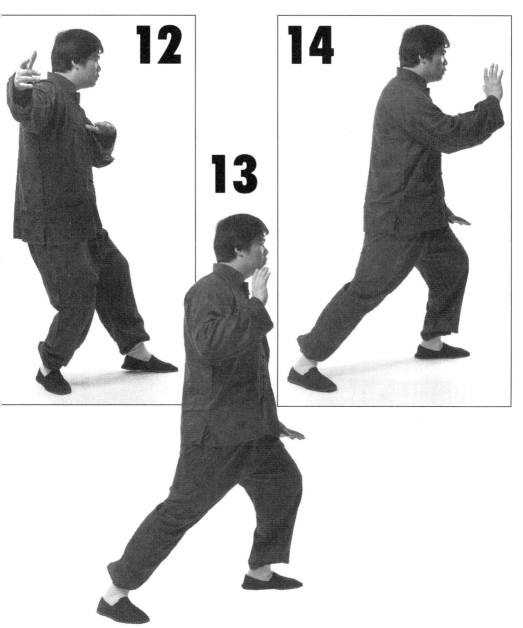

5. Brush Knee and Twist Step (right)

A. Turn your right wrist and drop your right hand down and out to the right side with your palms facing forward. Bring your left hand to your chest *(fig. 12)*.

B. Drop your left hand down swiftly to your left side with its palm facing downward, while bringing your right hand to your right shoulder with its palm facing forward *(fig. 13)*.

C. Push your right hand forward with its palm facing forward *(fig. 14)*.

43

6. Brush Knee and Twist Step (left)

A. Turn your left palm upward and bring your left hand to the left side with its palm facing forward. At the same time, bring your right hand up to your chest with its palm facing downward *(figs. 15, 16)*.

B. Turn the toes of your left foot outward, while stepping forward with your right foot *(figs. 17, 18)*. Move your right hand down beside your right knee, while bringing your left hand back to your left shoulder. From here, push your left arm forward with its palm facing forward *(fig. 19)*.

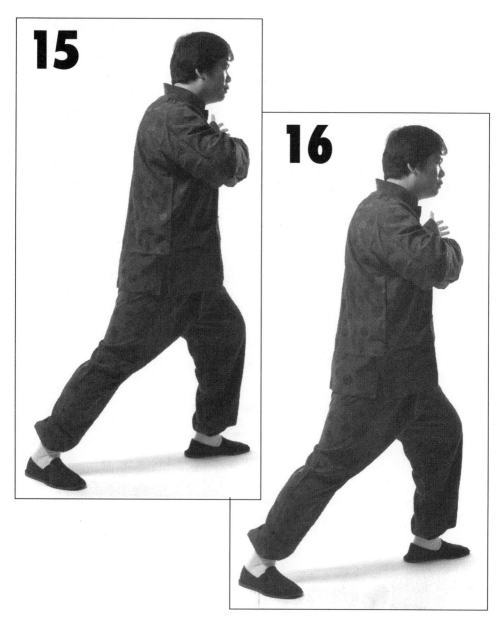

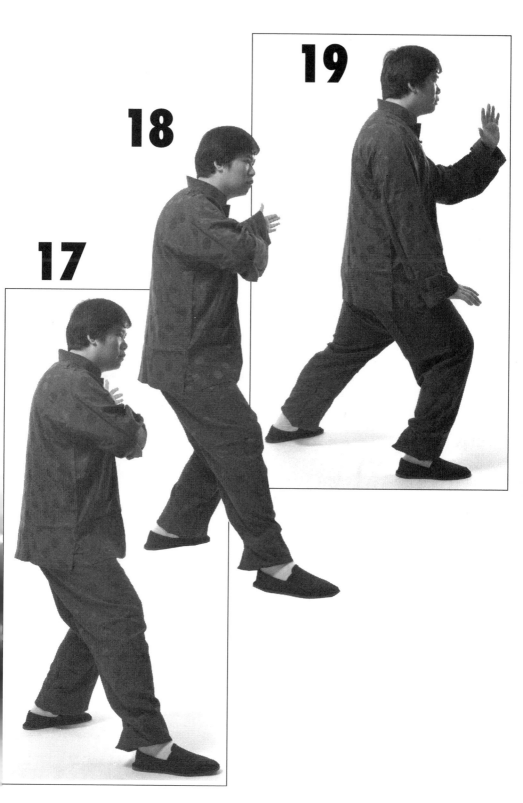

45

7. Brush Knee and Twist Step (right)

A. Turn your right palm until it faces upward, then bring your right hand to your right side, with its palm facing forward, and your left hand up to chest level, with its palm facing downward *(fig. 20)*.

B. Turn the toes of your right foot outward, while stepping forward with your left foot *(fig. 21)*. Lower your left hand to the side of your left knee while bringing your right hand back to your right shoulder, and then push forward with your right hand, with its palm facing forward *(fig. 22)*.

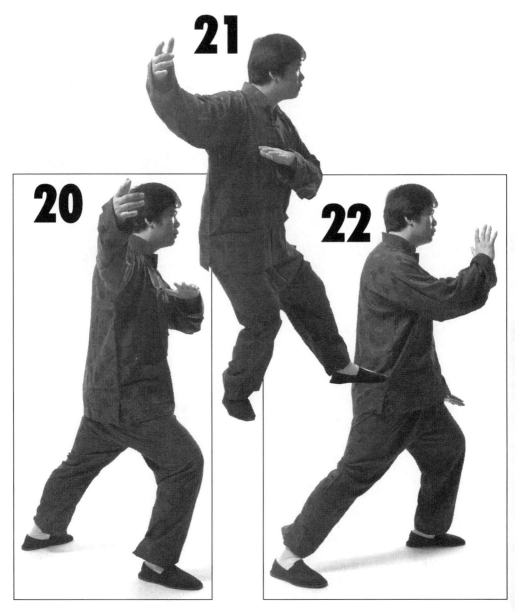

8. Fist Under Elbow

A. Clench your right hand into a fist and move your right foot a half-step closer to your foot *(fig. 23)*.

B. Slowly shift your body weight onto your right foot. Pull your right fist close to your chest and place the elbow of your left arm on top of your right fist *(fig. 24)*. Land on the heel of your left foot *(fig. 25)*.

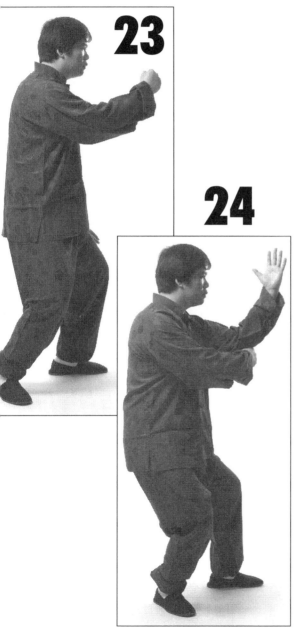

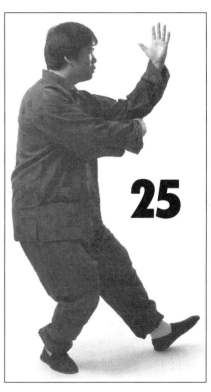

9. Step Backward and Drive Away Monkey (right)

A. Open your fist and carry your right hand to your right side with its palm facing forward *(figs. 26)*.

B. Extend your left hand straight with its palm facing upward *(fig. 27)*.

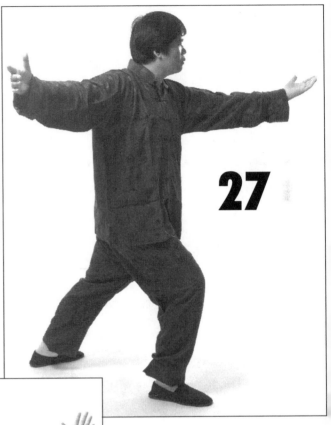

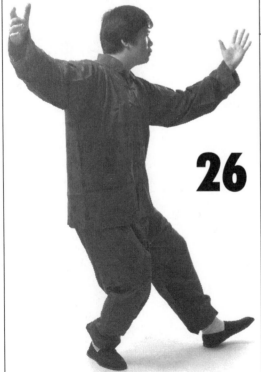

C. Step back with your left foot and then place your weight on it, then bring your right hand back to its shoulder *(fig. 28)*.

D. Push your right hand forward, with its palm facing forward, while bringing your left hand, with its palm facing upward, back to the left side of your hip *(fig. 29)*.

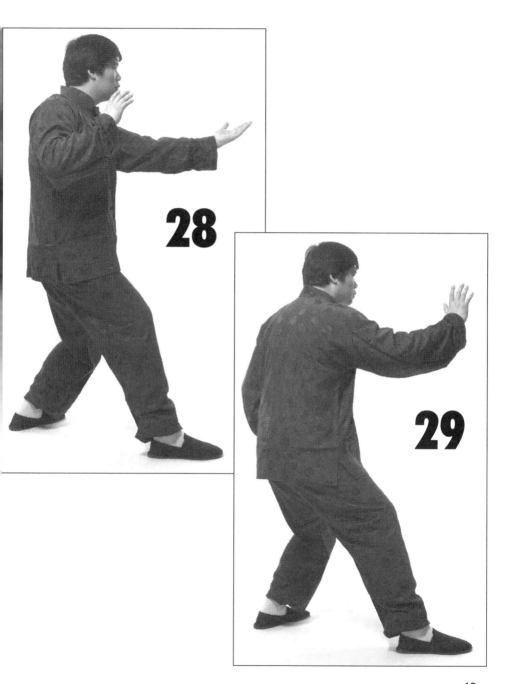

10. Step Backward and Drive Away Monkey (left)

A. Carry your left hand to the left side with its palm facing forward *(fig. 30)*.

A. Extend your right hand with its palm facing upward *(fig. 31)*.

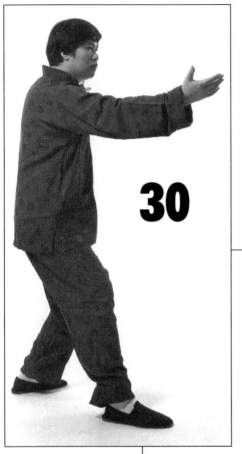

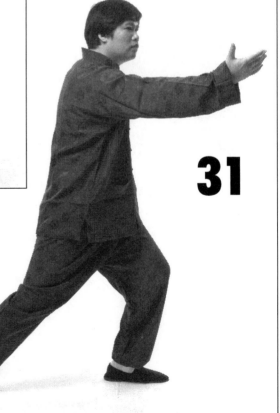

C. Step backward with your right foot and then place your weight on it, then bring your left hand back to your left shoulder *(fig. 32).*

D. Push your left hand forward with its palm facing forward, while bringing your right hand back to the right side of your hips with its palm facing upward *(fig. 33).*

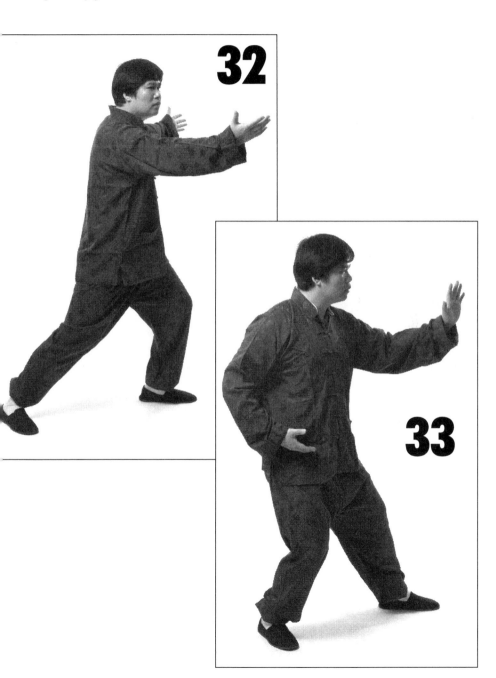

11. Step Backward and Drive Away Monkey (right)

A. Carry your right hand to the right side with its palm facing forward, while extending your left hand with its palm facing forward *(Fig. 34)*.

B. Step back with your left foot, placing your weight onto your right foot *(fig. 35)*.

C. Bring your right hand back to your right shoulder then push it forward with its palm face forward, while bringing your left hand back to the left side of your hips with its palm facing upward *(figs. 36, 37)*.

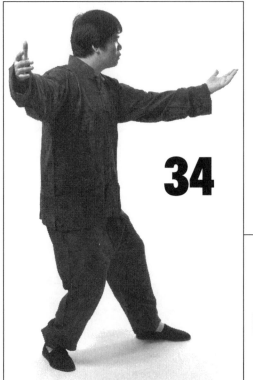

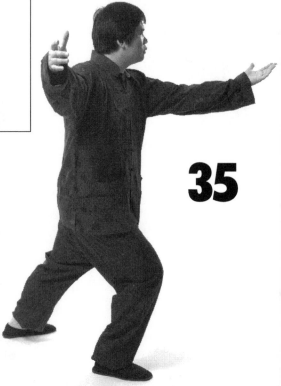

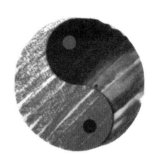

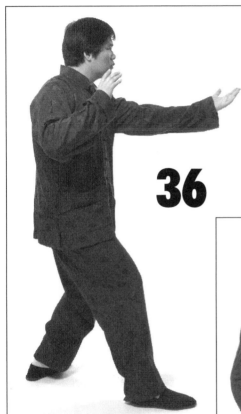

36

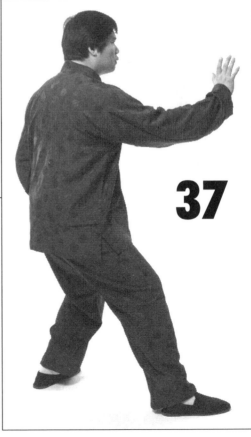

37

12. Step Backward and Drive Away Monkey (left)

A. Carry your left hand to the left side of your face with its palm facing forward *(fig. 38)*.

B. Extend your right hand straight with its palm facing upward. Step back with your right foot and then place your weight on it *(figs. 39-41)*.

C. Bring your left hand back to your left shoulder then push it forward with its palm facing forward, while bringing your right hand back to the right side of your hips with its palm facing upward. *(fig. 42.*

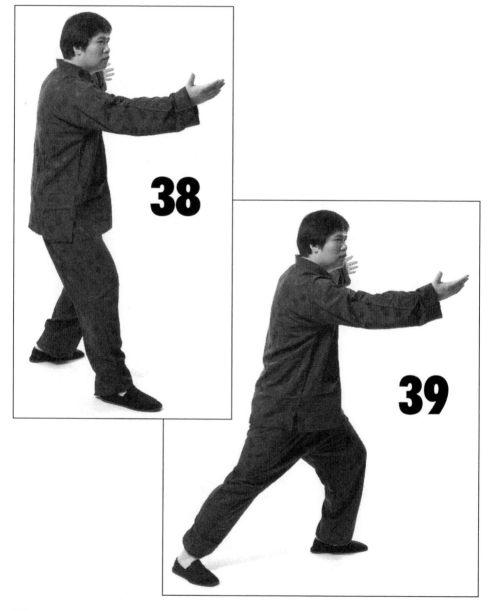

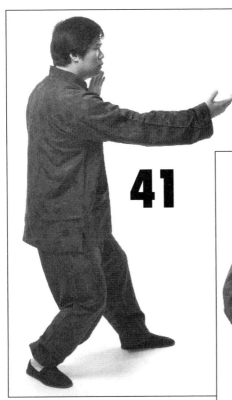

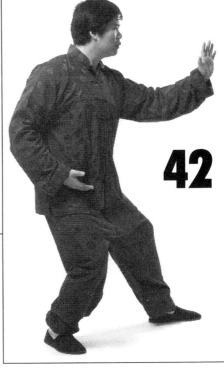

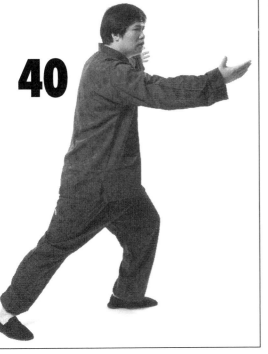

13. Grasp Sparrow's Tail (left)

A. Lift your right hand with its palm facing downward then bring your left hand, with its palm facing upward, under your right hand *(fig. 43)*. Follow this with the four primary tai chi chuan movements: Ward-off, Roll-back, Press, and Push.

B. Ward-off: Place your body weight onto your right foot and step forward with your left foot. Carry both hands in front of your chest with your left hand positioned outside of your right hand, but with both palms facing *(fig. 44)*.

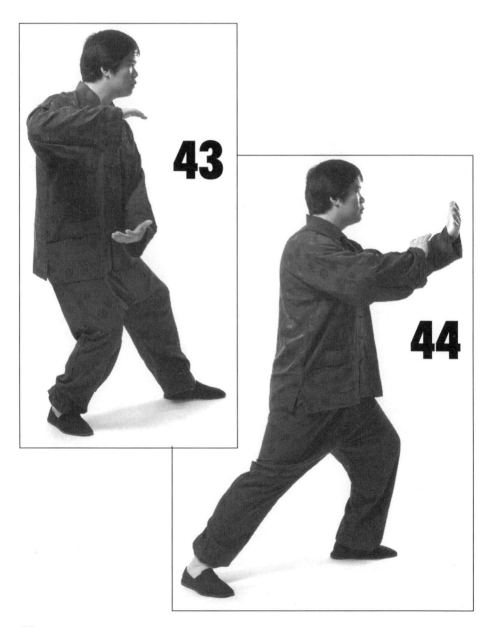

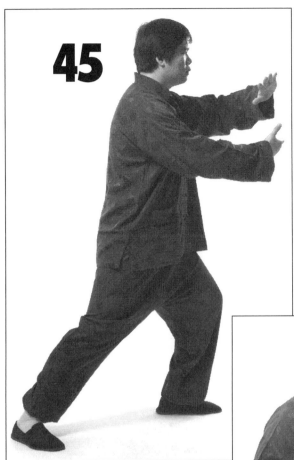

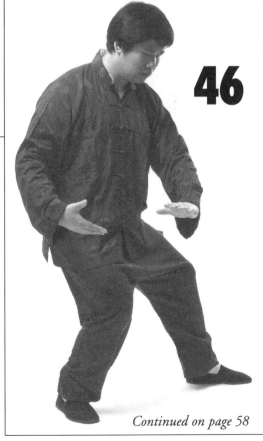

C. Roll-back: Turn your hands so that the palm of the right hand faces upward and the palm of the left hand faces downward. Simultaneously shift your body weight and move your hands to the right side of your hips *(figs. 45, 46)*.

Continued on page 58

13. Grasp Sparrow's Tail (left)
Continued from page 57

D. Press: Turn your left hand until its palm faces upward, then push your right hand against your left wrist. Simultaneously shift your body weight onto your left foot while pushing both hands out *(figs. 47, 48)*.

E. Push: Open both hands with the palms facing downward and then bring your hands back to your chest. From here, turn your palms until they face outwards and then push both hands out *(figs. 49–52)*.

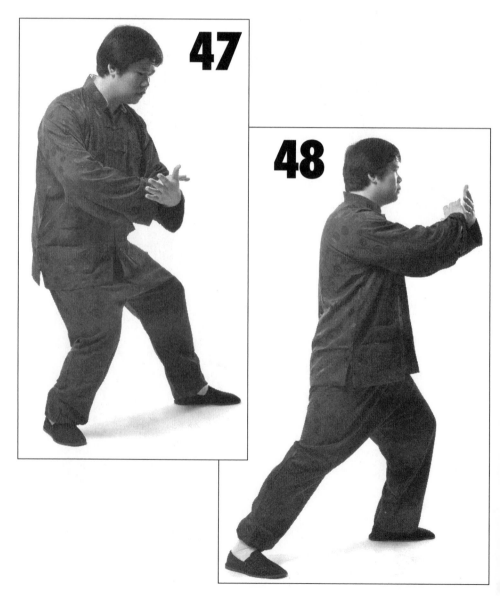

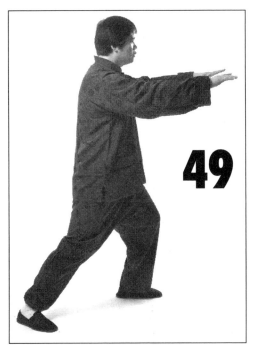

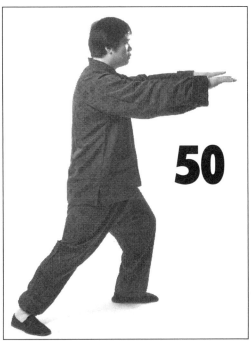

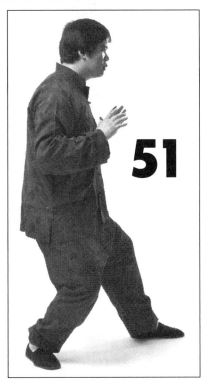

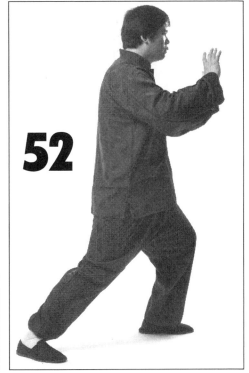

14. Grasp Sparrow's Tail (right)

A. Bring both hands back to your body with the weight onto your right foot, then simultaneously turn your left foot, body, and your hands to the right corner *(figs. 53, 54)*. Follow this with the four primary tai chi chuan movements: Ward-off, Roll-back, Press, and Push.

B. Ward-Off: After the turn, shift your body weight onto your left foot. Your left hand will remain on top with its palm facing downward while bringing your right hand under your left hand, with its palms facing upward *(fig. 55)*.

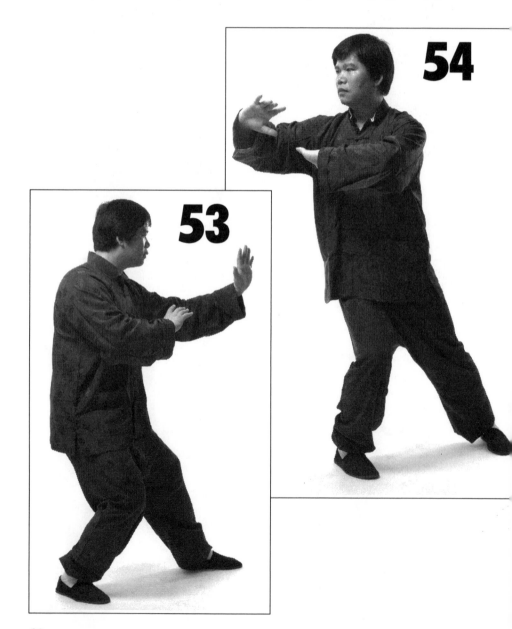

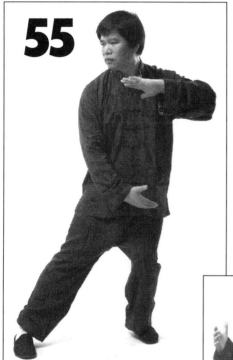

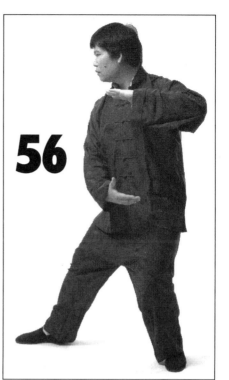

C. Roll Back: Step forward with your right foot, placing your body weight on it. Carry both hands in front of your chest, with your right hand outside your left hand (*figs. 56, 57*).

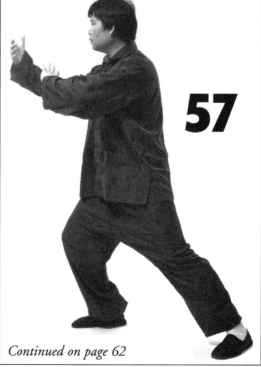

Continued on page 62

14. Grasp Sparrow's Tail (right)

Continued from page 61

D. Press: Turn the left palm to face upward and the right palm to face downward. Simultaneously, shift your body weight and hands to the left side of your hip *(figs. 58–60)*.

E. Push: Turn your right hand to upward and then push against the right wrist with your left hand. Simultaneously shift your body weight onto your right foot and push both hands out *(fig. 61)*.

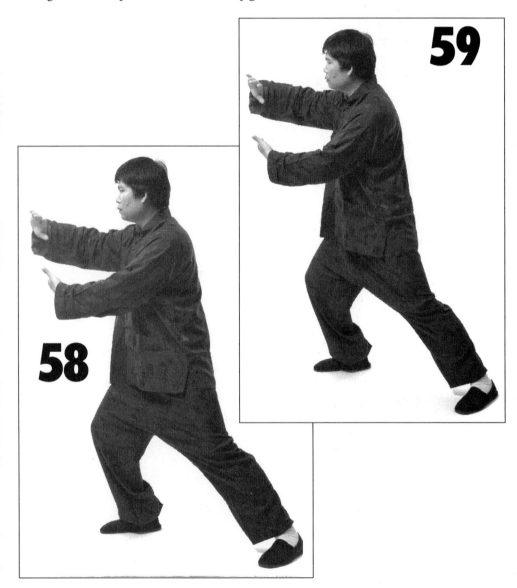

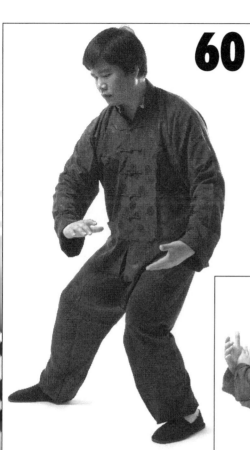

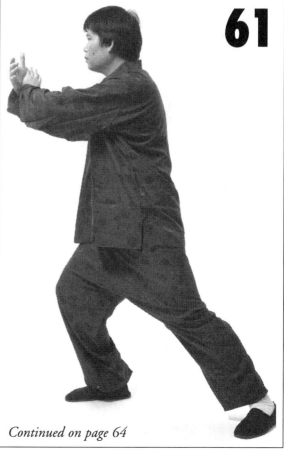

Continued on page 64

14. Grasp Sparrow's Tail (right)

Continued from page 63

F. Open both hands with their palms facing downward, then bring the hands back to your chest. Turn the palms to face outward and push both hands out *(figs. 62–65)*.

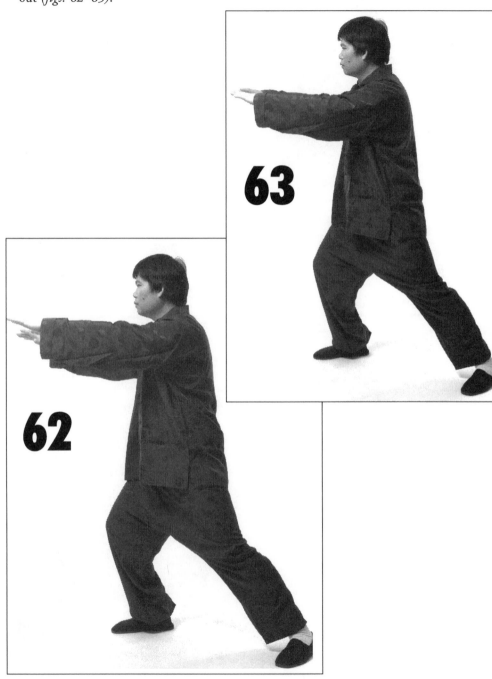

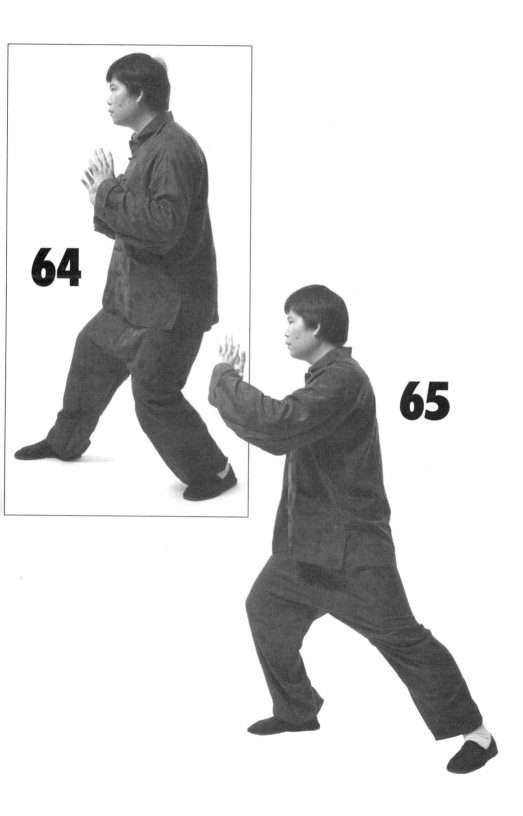

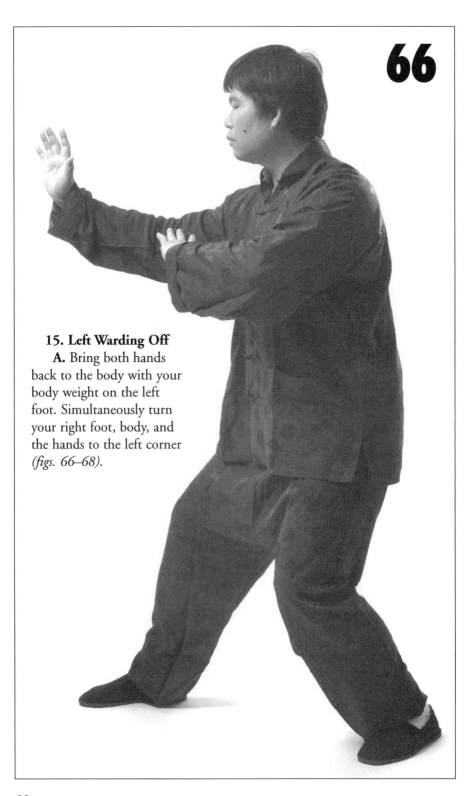

15. Left Warding Off

A. Bring both hands back to the body with your body weight on the left foot. Simultaneously turn your right foot, body, and the hands to the left corner *(figs. 66–68).*

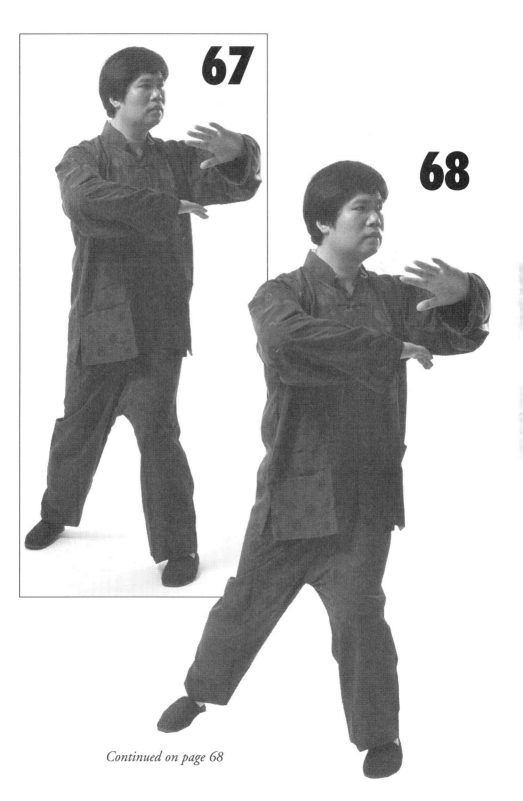

Continued on page 68

15. Left Warding Off
Continued from page 67

B. After the turn, shift the body weight back onto your right foot with your right hand remaining on top with the palms facing downward. Bring your left hand under your right hand, with its palm facing upward *(fig. 69)*.

C. Step forward with your left foot and place your the body weight on it. Lift your left hand up with its palm facing inward and push your right hand down to your right leg *(figs. 70–72)*.

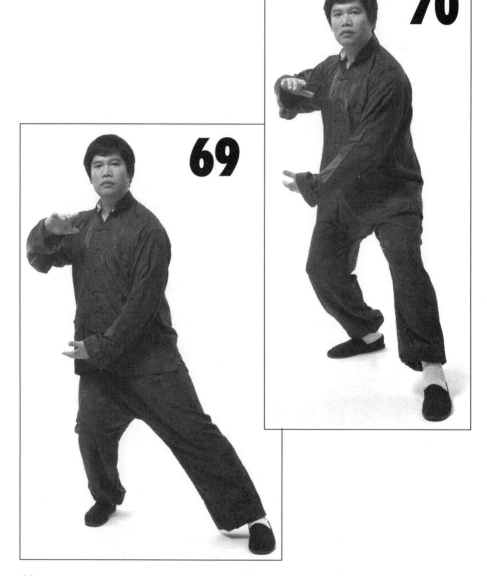

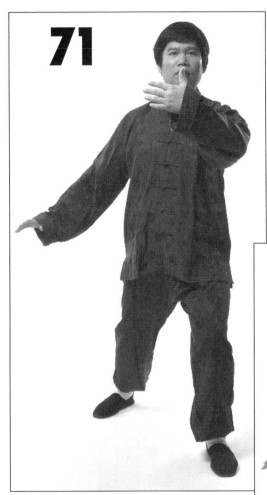

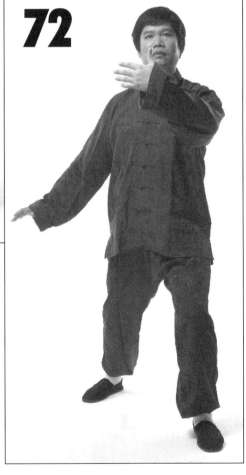

16. Wave Hands Like Clouds (5 times)

A. Bring your right hand to your left knee then exchange your hands with the right hand up and the left hand down *(fig. 73)*.

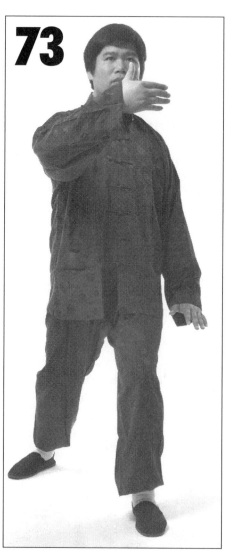

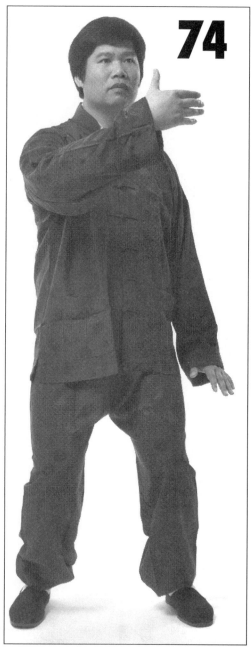

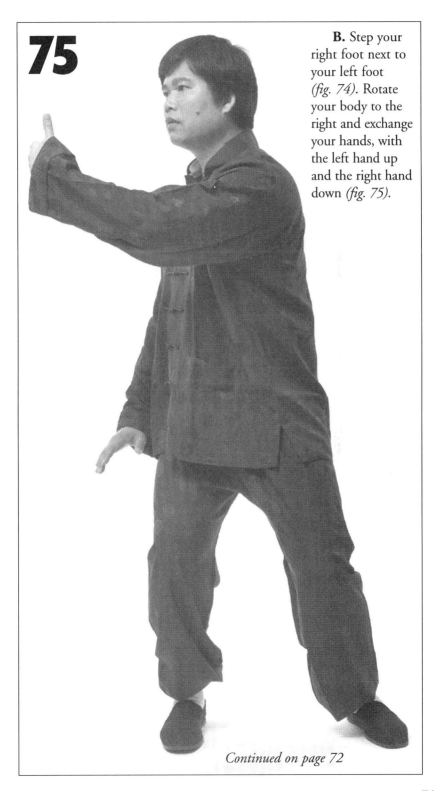

75

B. Step your right foot next to your left foot *(fig. 74)*. Rotate your body to the right and exchange your hands, with the left hand up and the right hand down *(fig. 75)*.

Continued on page 72

16. Wave Hands Like Clouds
(5 times)

Continued from page 71

C. Step to the left with your left foot then shift your body weight onto your left foot and rotate the body to the left side and exchange the hands with the right hand up and the left hand down *(fig. 76)*.

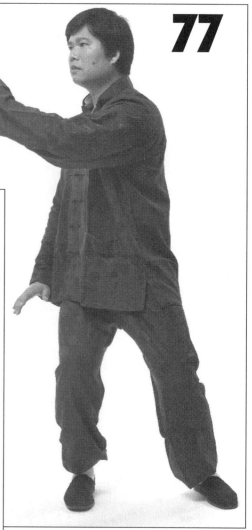

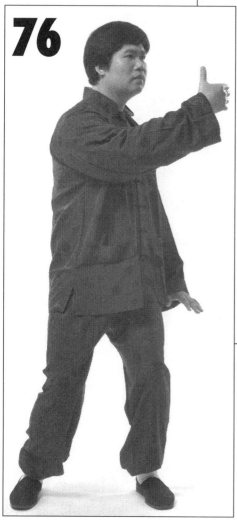

D. Step your right foot next to your left foot. Simultaneously shift your body weight onto your right foot and rotate your body to the right side and exchange the hands with your left hand up and your right hand down *(fig. 77)*.

78

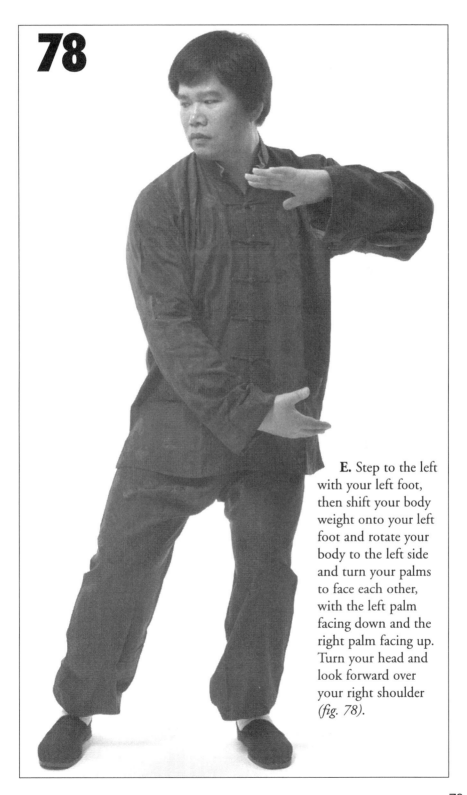

E. Step to the left with your left foot, then shift your body weight onto your left foot and rotate your body to the left side and turn your palms to face each other, with the left palm facing down and the right palm facing up. Turn your head and look forward over your right shoulder *(fig. 78)*.

17. Fair Lady Works on Shuttles (right)

A. With the body weight on your left foot, rotate your body to the right. Pick up your right foot and step 45 degrees to the right *(fig. 79)*.

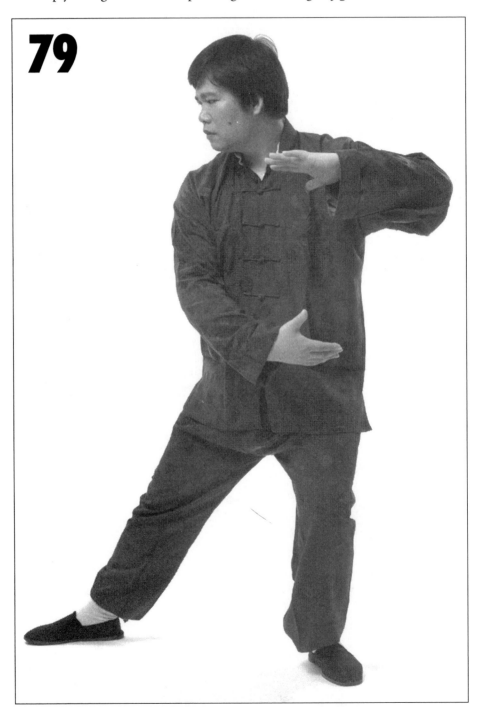

79

B. Slowly shift your body weight onto your right foot. Set your right hand above your head and push your left hand forward from the left shoulder *(fig. 80)*.

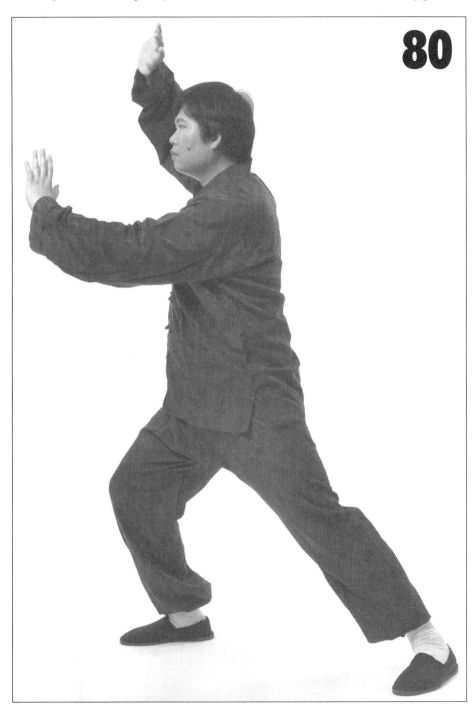

18. Turn Around and Chop

A. Turn your left hand with its palm facing up *(fig. 81)*. Slowly shift your body weight back onto your left foot, while at the same time pulling both hands down to the left side of your hips, with the right hand clenched into a fist *(fig. 82)*.

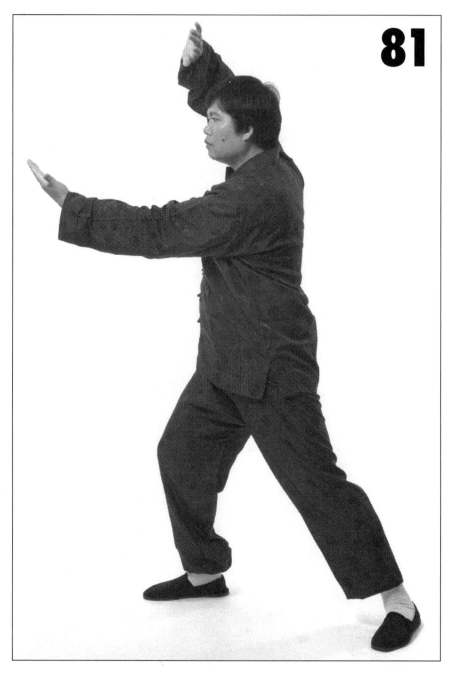

81

B. With your body weight on your left foot, pick up your right foot and then step forward, with the toes pointing to the corner *(fig. 83)*.

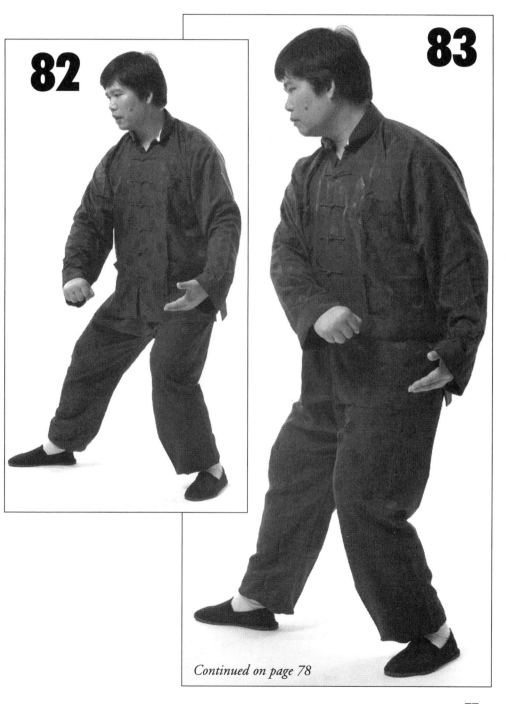

Continued on page 78

18. Turn Around and Chop

Continued from page 77

C. Make a fist circle to the right around your body, resting on the right side of your hip, then push your left hand forward *(figs. 84–86)*.

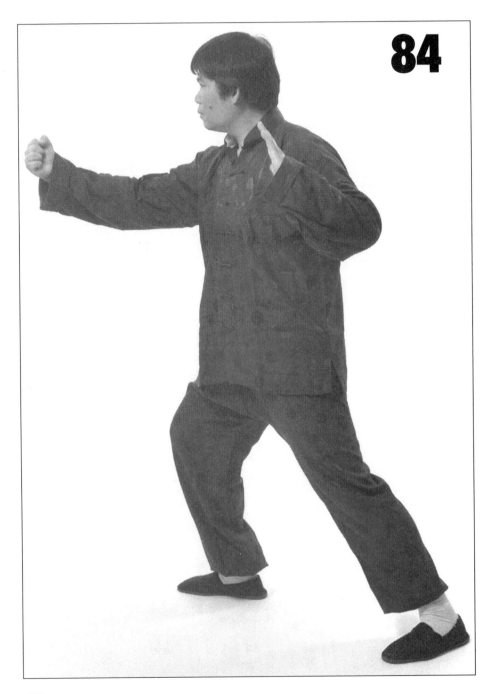

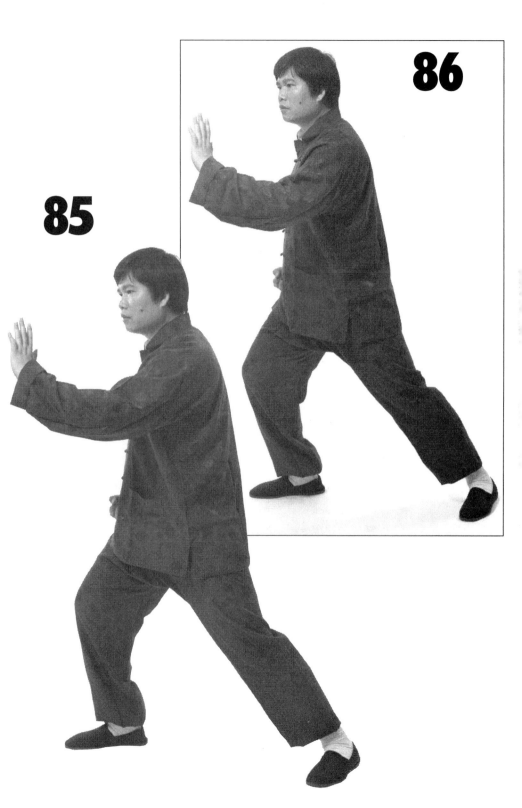

19. Step Forward and Punch

A. Step forward with your left foot, and place your body weight on it upon setting it down. Punch forward with your right hand *(figs. 87, 88)*.

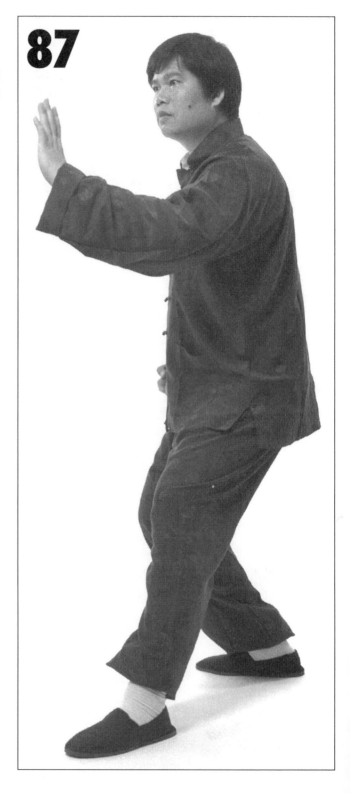

87

88

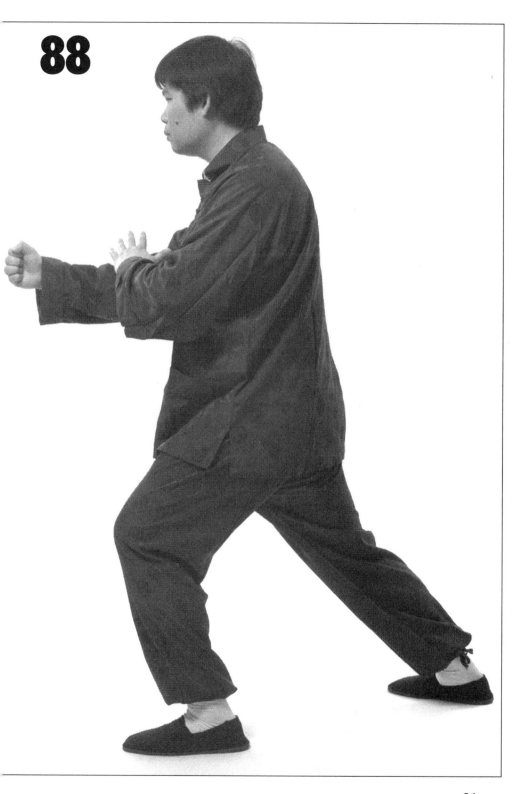

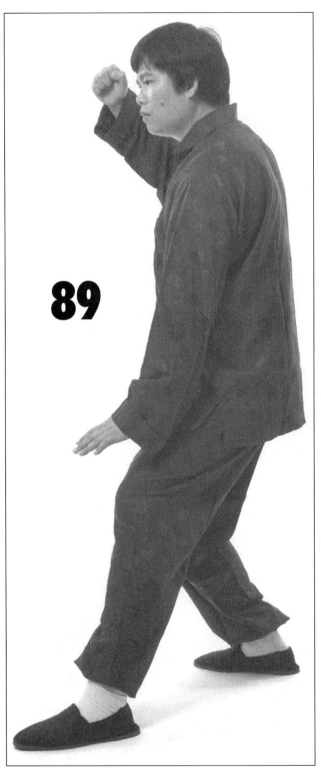

89

20. Wild Horse Ruffling Its Mane (left)

A. Shift your body weight back onto your right foot. Simultaneously separate your hands with your right fist going up to your right ear and your left palm pushing down to your left knee *(fig. 89)*.

B. Turn your left palm to face up and open your right fist at chest level, with the palms facing each other *(fig. 90)*.

C. Turn the toes of your left foot outward. Slowly shift your body weight onto your left foot, while at the same time separating your hands so that your left hand moves up and your right hand moves down *(fig. 91)*.

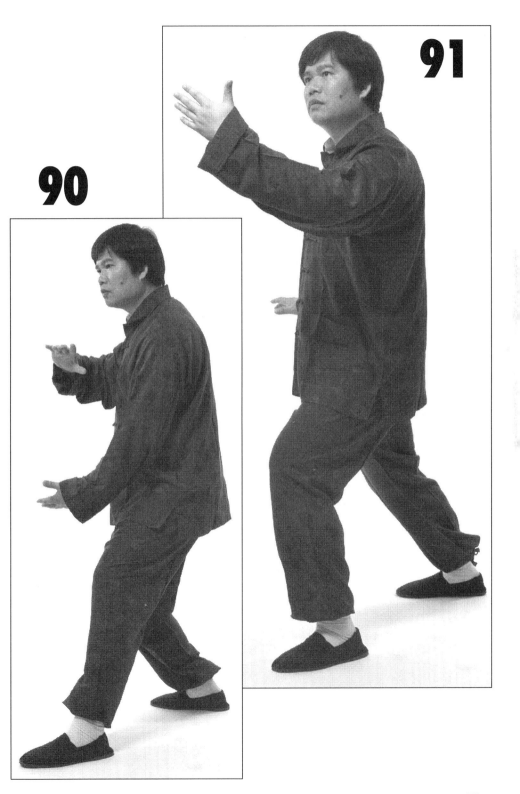

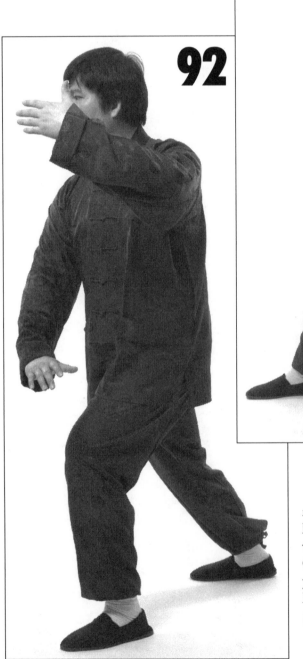

21. Grasp Sparrow's Tail (right)

A. Ward-Off: Move your right hand to face your left knee *(fig. 92)*, then step forward with your right foot. Carry both hands in front of your chest, with your right hand outside your left hand *(figs. 93, 94)*.

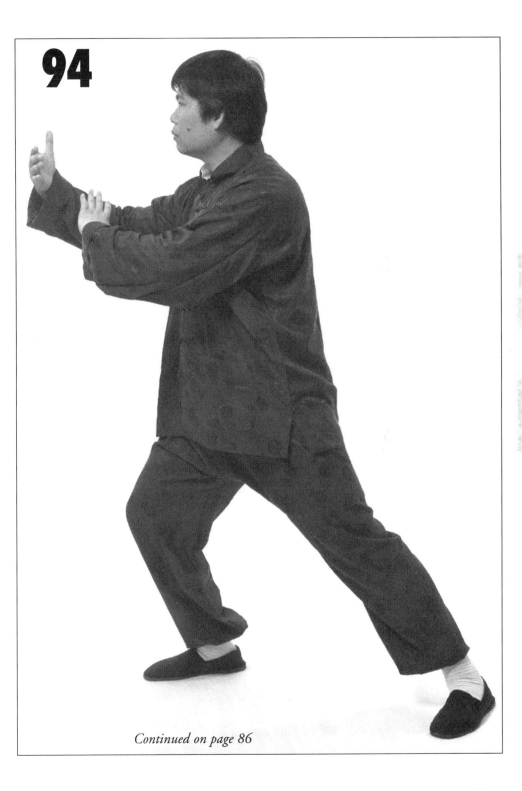

94

Continued on page 86

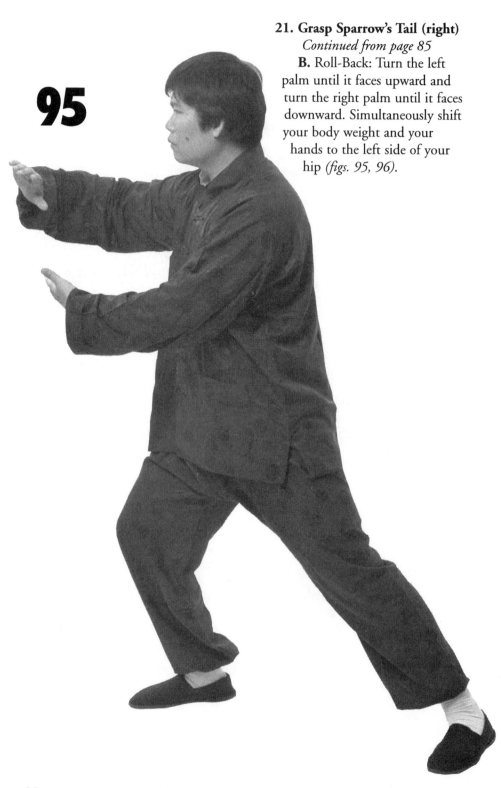

95

21. Grasp Sparrow's Tail (right)
Continued from page 85
B. Roll-Back: Turn the left palm until it faces upward and turn the right palm until it faces downward. Simultaneously shift your body weight and your hands to the left side of your hip *(figs. 95, 96).*

C. Press: Turn your right hand to face upward and then push your left hand against your right wrist. Simultaneously shift your body weight onto your right foot and push both hands out *(fig. 97).*

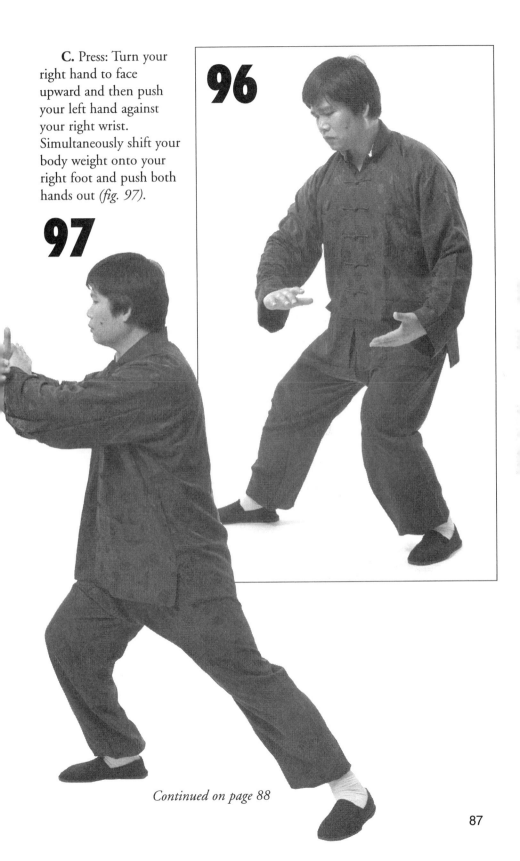

Continued on page 88

21. Grasp Sparrow's Tail (right)

Continued from page 87

D. Push: Open both hands with their palm facing downward, then bring the hands back to your chest. Turn your palms until they face outward and then push both hands out *(figs. 98-100)*.

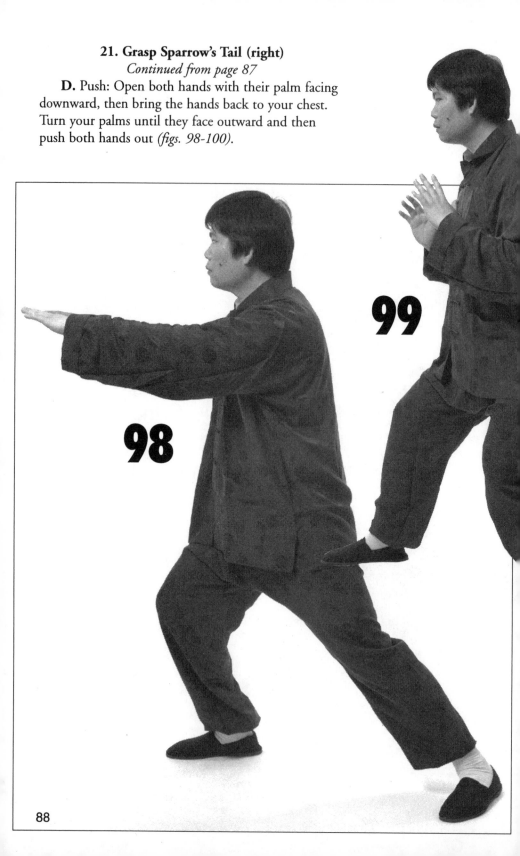

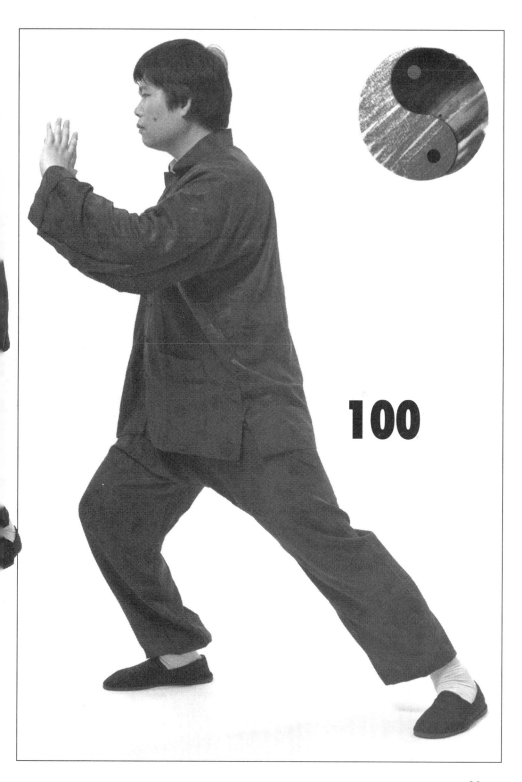

100

22. Closing Tai Chi Chuan

A. Bring both hands back to your chest, with your body weight on your left foot *(fig. 101)*.

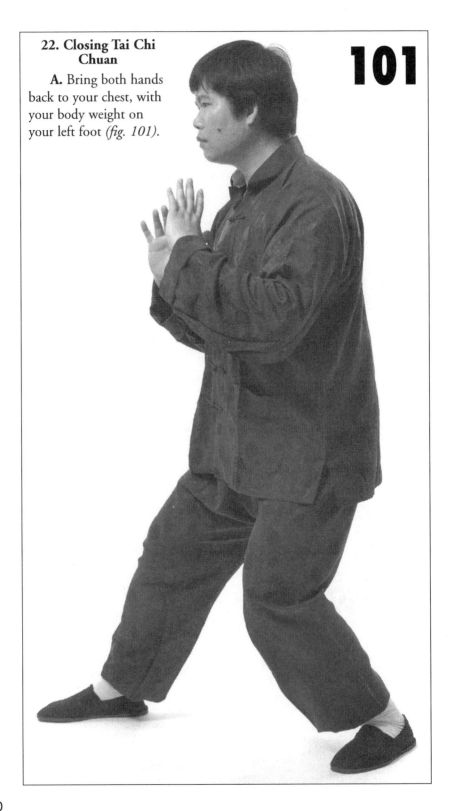

101

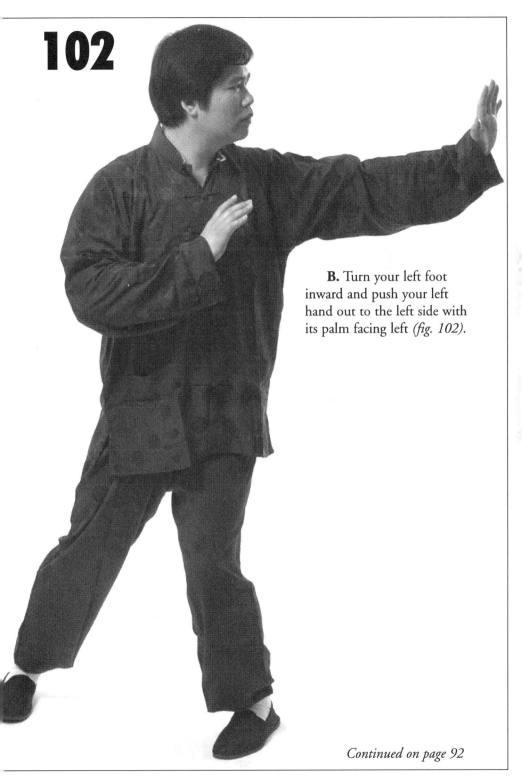

102

B. Turn your left foot inward and push your left hand out to the left side with its palm facing left *(fig. 102)*.

Continued on page 92

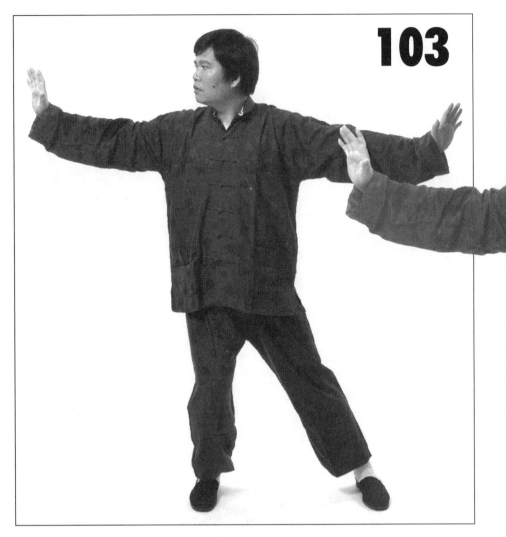

22. Closing Tai Chi Chuan
Continued from page 87

C. Keeping your left hand where it is, shift your body weight onto your right foot and push your right hand to the right with its palm facing the right *(fig. 103)*. Step your left foot next to your right foot with your hands held level to shoulder level *(fig. 104)*.

D. Bring both hands down to the area between your knees, with the hands crossing right under left *(fig. 105)*.

104

105

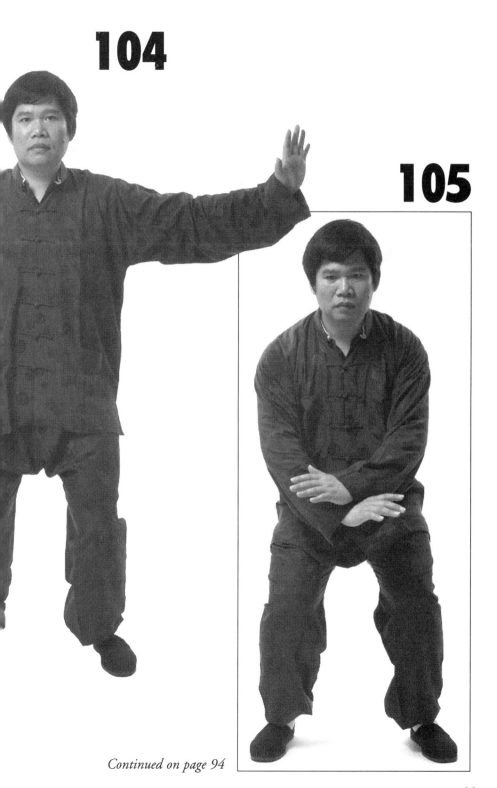

Continued on page 94

106 107

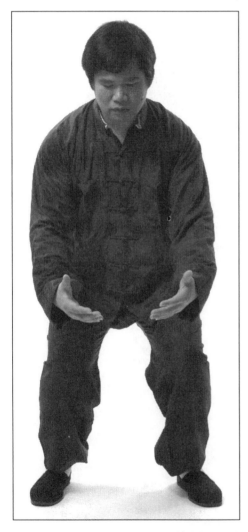 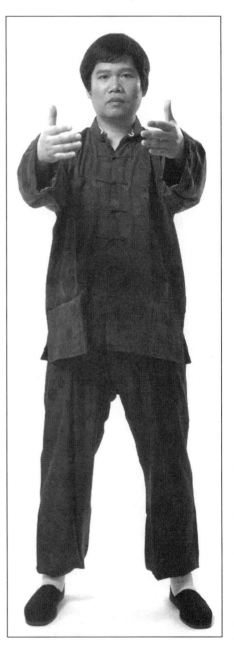

22. Closing Tai Chi Chuan
Continued from page 93

    E. Turn your hands to face upward, separate them, and bring them up to the shoulders, with the palms facing each other *(figs. 106, 107)*.

108   109

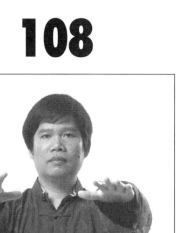
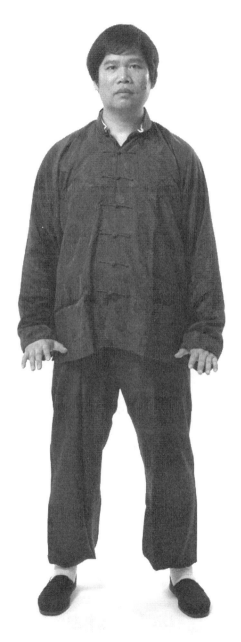

Continued on page 96

F. Turn your palms to face downward, drop your hands down to each side of your legs *(figs. 108-109)*.

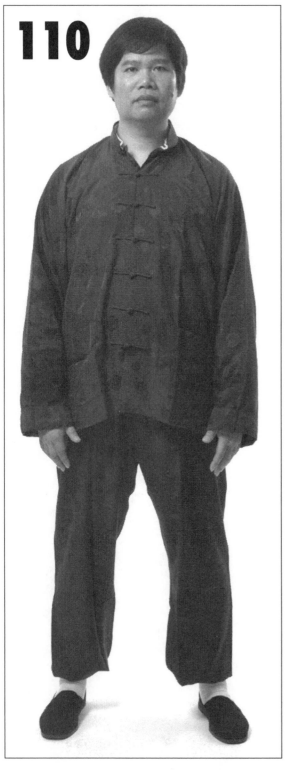

110

22. Closing Tai Chi Chuan
Continued from page 95

End, return to start position, with both feet pointing forward and held firmly to the ground a shoulders-width apart. The knees are held together loosely. The hands are held relaxed down along the sides of their respective legs *(fig. 110)*.

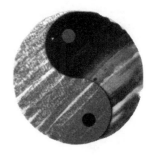

THE 22-TECHNIQUE YANG STYLE FORM

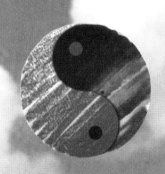

THE 22-TECHNIQUE YANG STYLE FORM

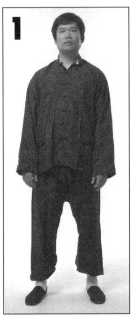

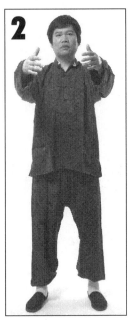

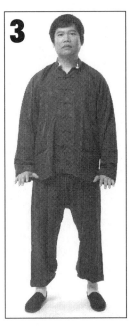

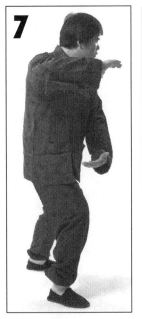

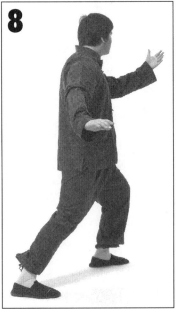

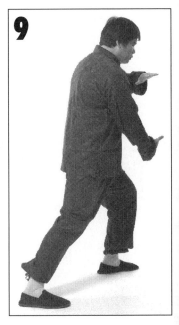

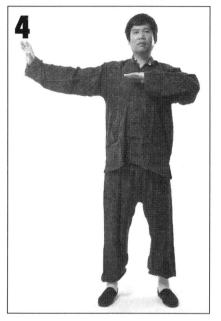
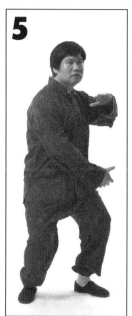
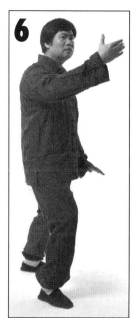
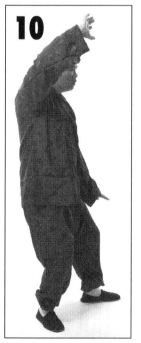
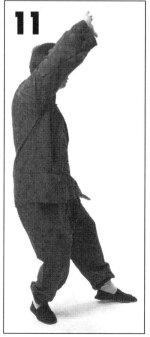
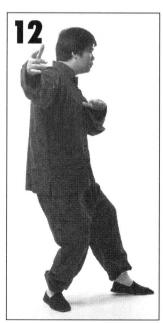

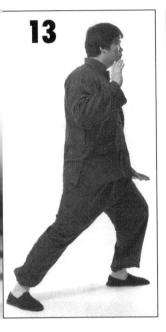
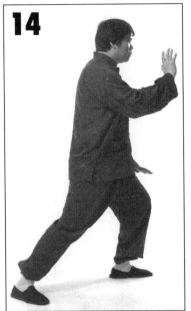
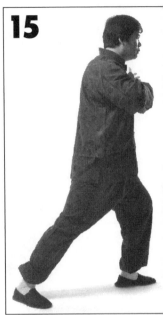

THE 22-TECHNIQUE YANG STYLE FORM

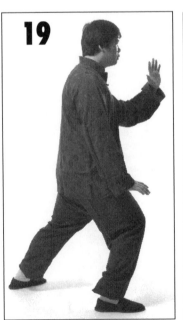
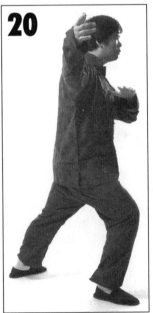
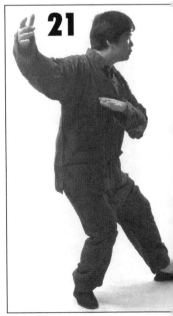

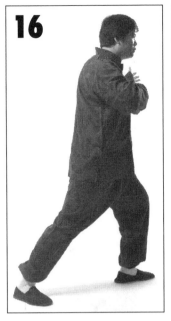 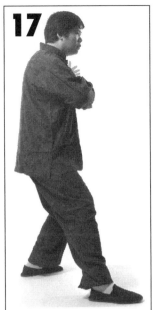 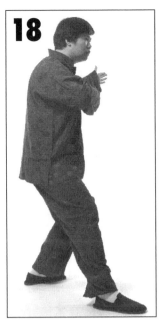

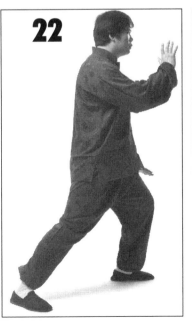 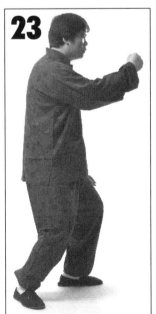 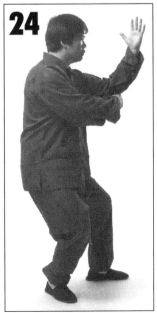

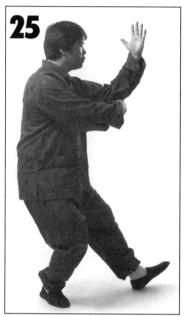 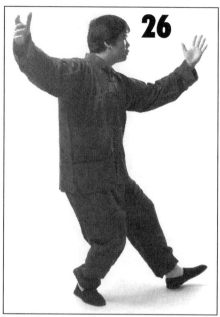

THE 22-TECHNIQUE YANG STYLE FORM

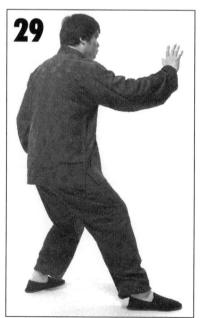 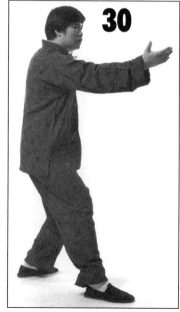

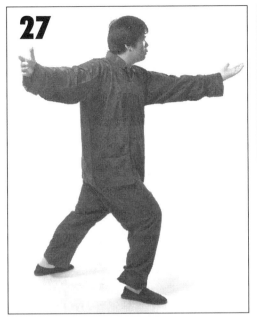

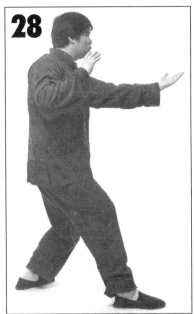

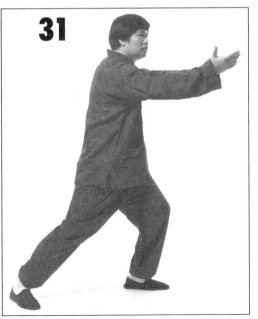

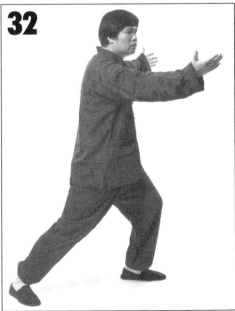

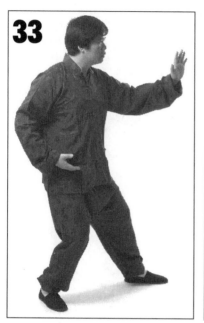
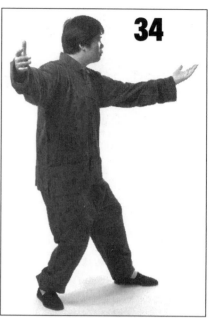

THE 22-TECHNIQUE YANG STYLE FORM

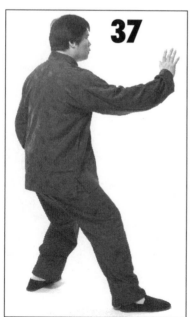
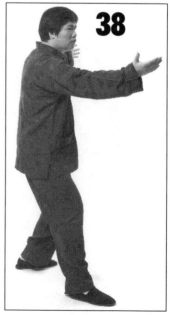

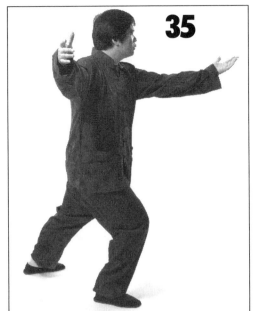
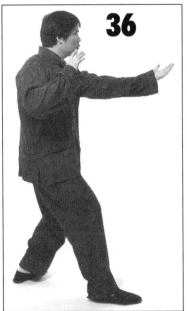

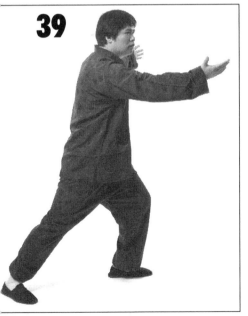
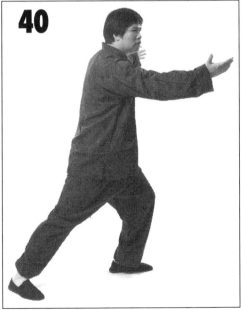

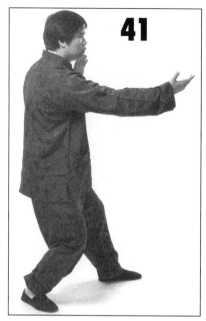
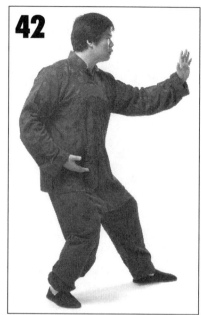

THE 22-TECHNIQUE YANG STYLE FORM

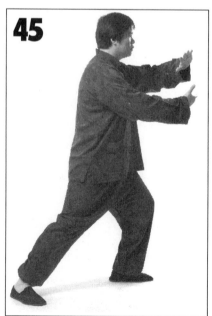
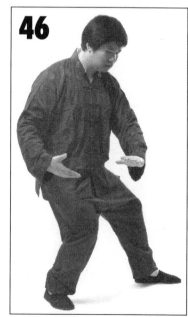

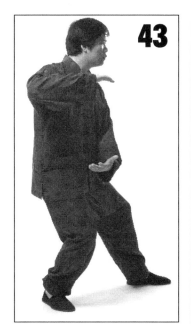

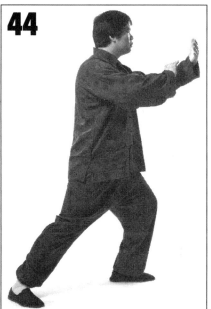

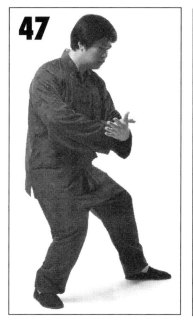

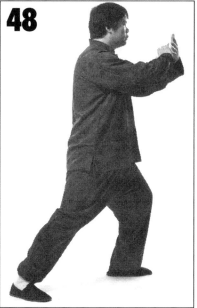

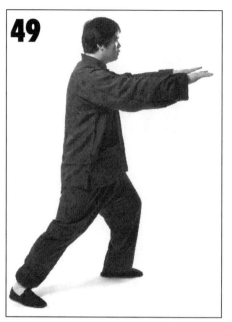

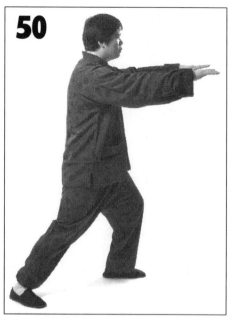

THE 22-TECHNIQUE YANG STYLE FORM

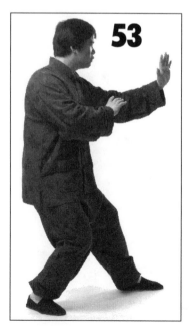

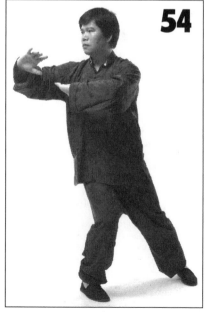

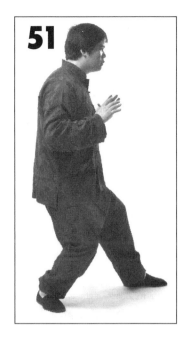

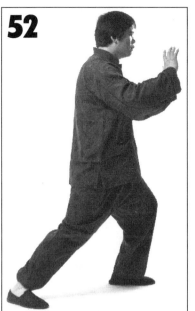

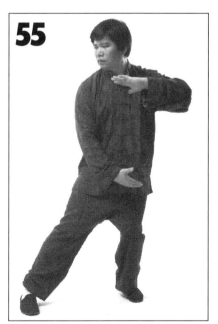

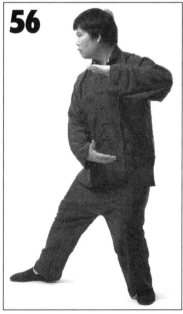

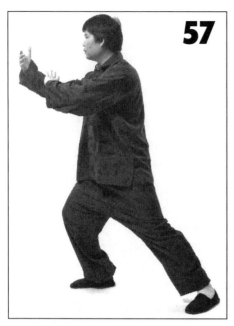

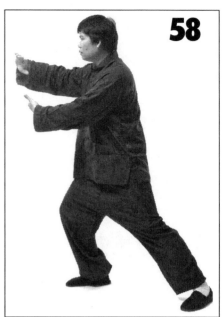

THE 22-TECHNIQUE YANG STYLE FORM

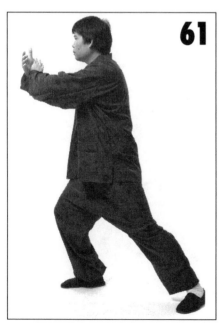

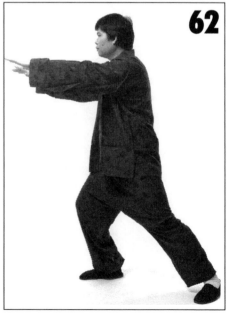

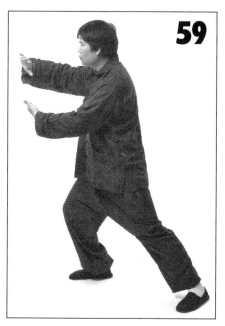 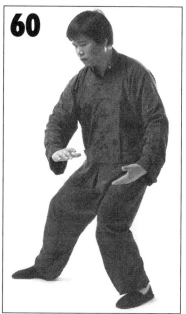

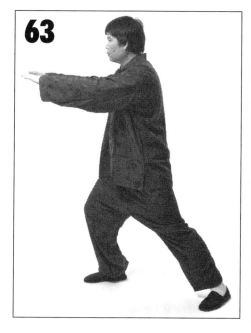 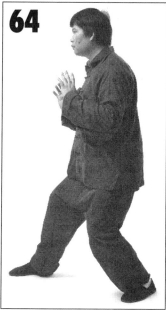

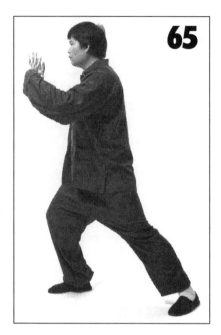 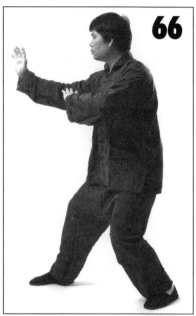

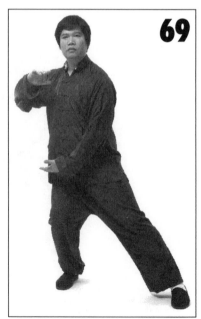 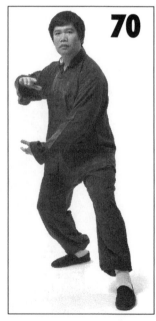

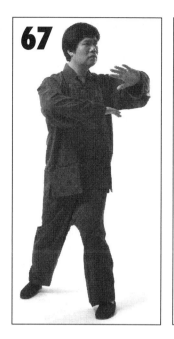

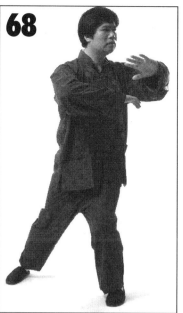

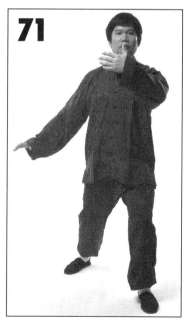

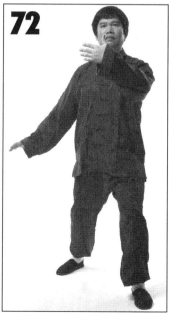

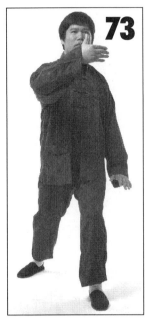 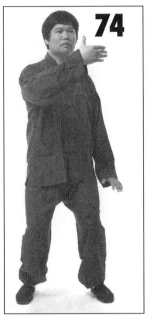 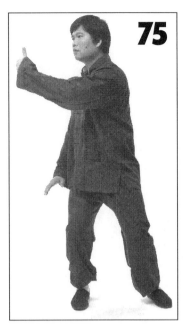

THE 22-TECHNIQUE YANG STYLE FORM

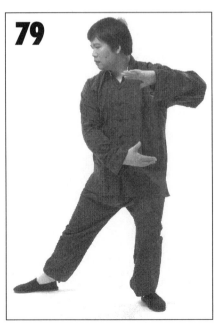 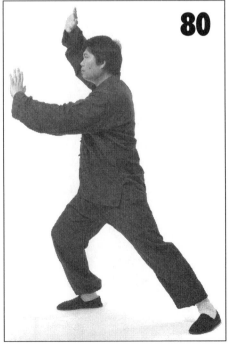

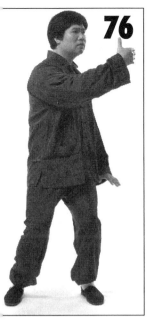
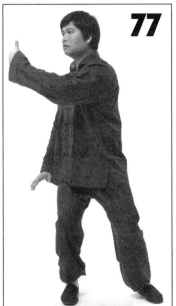
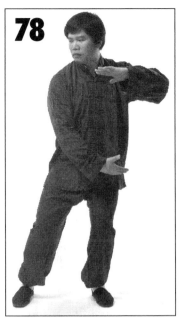

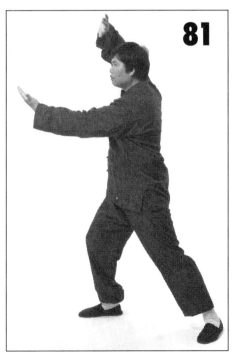
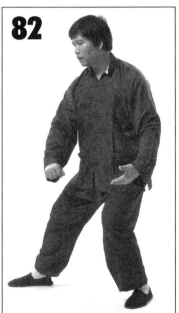

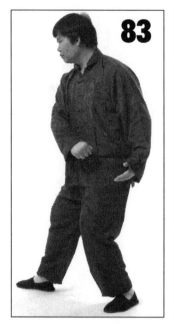
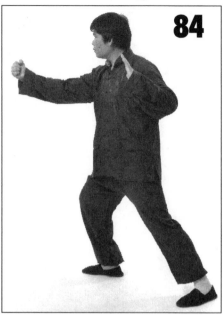

THE 22-TECHNIQUE YANG STYLE FORM

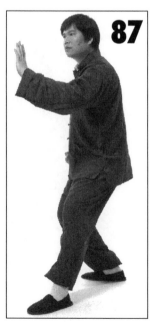
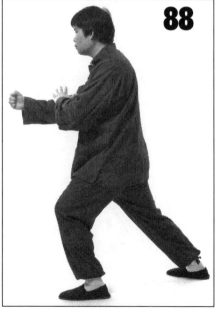

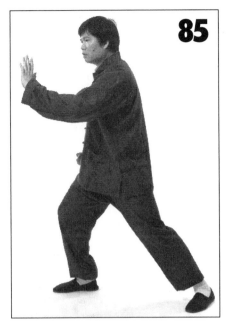
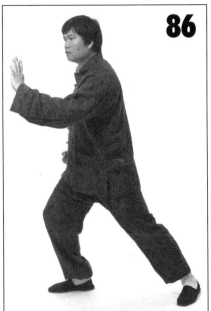

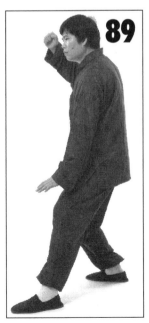
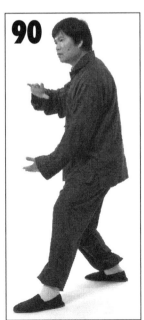
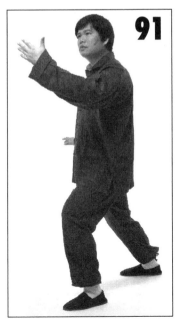

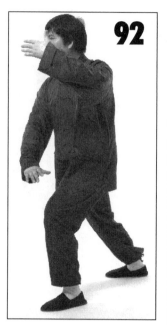 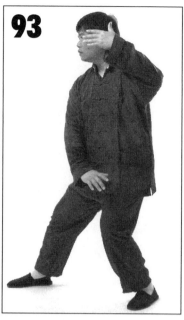

THE 22-TECHNIQUE YANG STYLE FORM

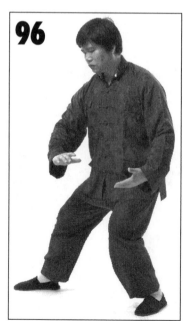 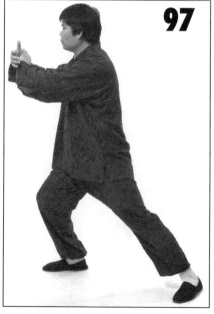

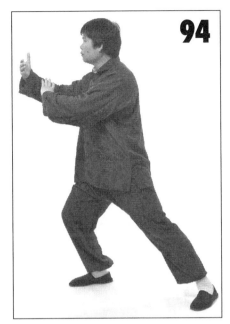

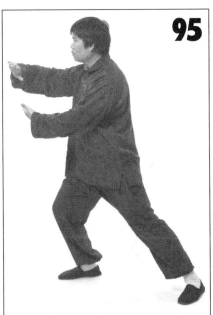

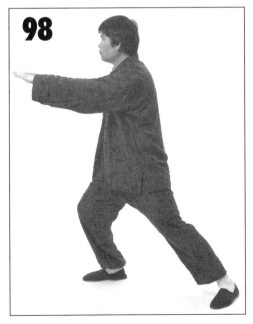

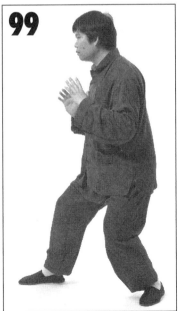

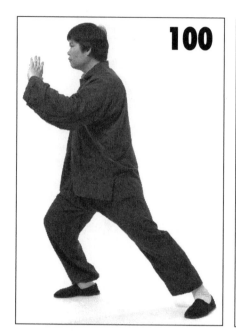
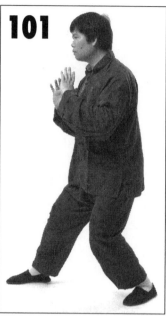

THE 22-TECHNIQUE YANG STYLE FORM

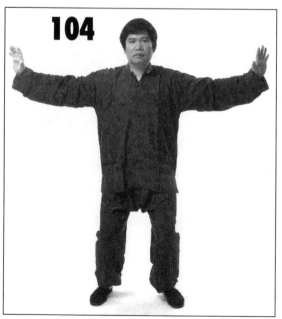
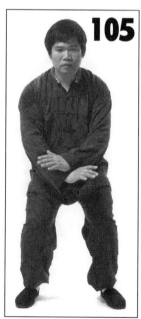

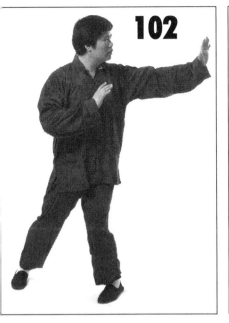

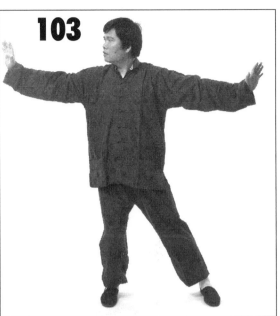

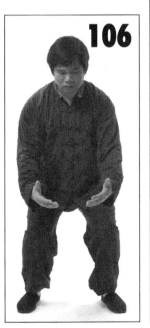

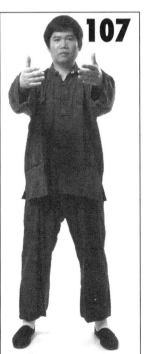

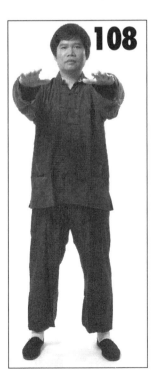

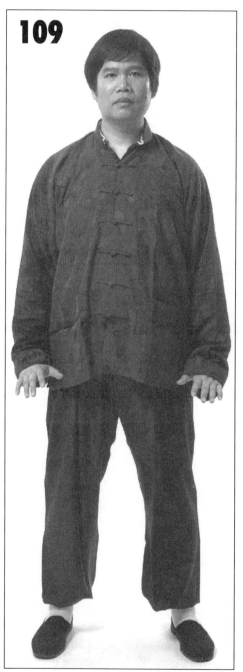

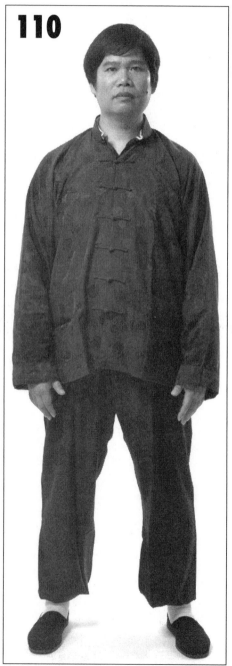

QUESTIONS & ANSWERS

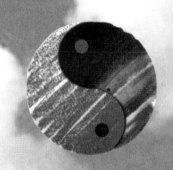

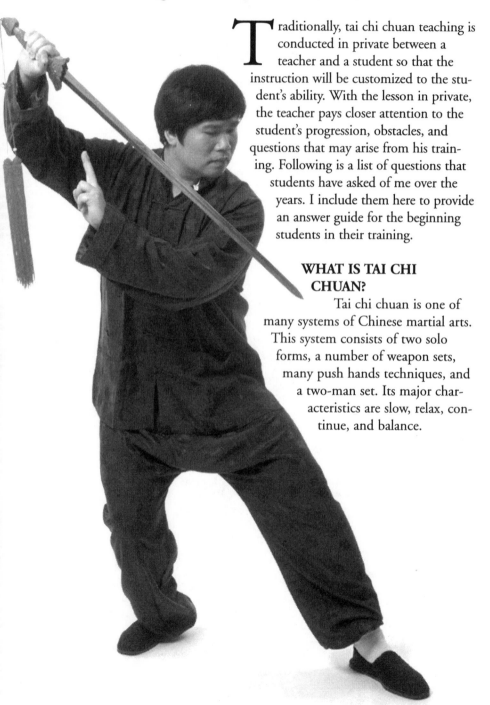

Chapter 8

QUESTIONS & ANSWERS

Traditionally, tai chi chuan teaching is conducted in private between a teacher and a student so that the instruction will be customized to the student's ability. With the lesson in private, the teacher pays closer attention to the student's progression, obstacles, and questions that may arise from his training. Following is a list of questions that students have asked of me over the years. I include them here to provide an answer guide for the beginning students in their training.

WHAT IS TAI CHI CHUAN?

Tai chi chuan is one of many systems of Chinese martial arts. This system consists of two solo forms, a number of weapon sets, many push hands techniques, and a two-man set. Its major characteristics are slow, relax, continue, and balance.

The solo form is composed of 13 principles: ward-off, roll back, press, push, pull down, elbows strike, shoulders strike, look to the left, look to the right, advance, retreat, and center. Each movement in the solo form is based on these 13 principles and must execute the mind, *chi* (internal energy), and power as one unit. This means that when the mind is focused on a specific area of the body, the *chi* will flow into that area. When the *chi* flows into an area, power will follow.

WHAT ARE THE 13 PRINCIPLE?

Tai chi chuan's 13 principles are divided into three segments: four direct gates, four corner gates, and five elements. The four direct gates are the movements of ward-off, roll back, press, and push. The four corner gates are the movements of pull down, split, elbows strike, and shoulders strike. These eight principles are called gates because they relate to the eight hexagrams in the *pa kua* diagram. The five elements are look to the left, look to the right, advance step, retreat step, and body equilibrium. These concepts are so-called after their formation of the five elements: fire, wood, water, metal, and earth.

WHAT IS YIN/YANG?

The term *yin/yang* was commonly used in ancient China as a general term for many things in life. It refers to two components which oppose each other and yet need each other for perfection. In tai chi chuan movements, *yin/yang* refers to some of the following terms: top vs. bottom; inside vs. outside; left vs. right; advance vs. retreat; and empty vs. full.

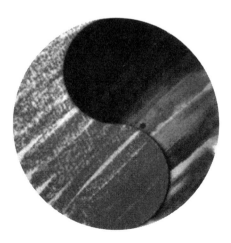

WHERE IS THE YIN/YANG IN TAI CHI CHUAN?

The *yin/yang* is referred to everywhere in the solo form. We can see it in the empty and full of the body weight; the open and close of each movement; the release and storing of the power; the up and down of the hands and body movements; the advance and retreat of the stepping; and the in and out of the breathing.

From this we can see that one should not focus on one area of the form but treat each movement as a whole in order to perfect the solo form. *Yin/yang* is the term referring to the whole, not its parts.

Let's take the movement "brush knee and twist step," for example. The first hand pushing forward is *yang* and the second hand brushing down to the knee is *yin*. If one understands the term *yin/yang*, one will not push the hand too far forward, which can cause the body lean too much. From an understanding of this term, one will maintain the correct posture at all times.

IS IT GOOD TO EMPHASIZE YIN/YANG IN TAI CHI CHUAN PRACTICE?

When this happens, one is emphasizing too much on the whole. A good whole begins with its individual parts. In order to perfect the solo form, one must practice each individual item as listed above. That is, mastering the empty and full will improve ones mobility; mastering the open and close will improve one in practical application, and so on.

WHY DO WE BEGIN WITH SLOW MOVEMENTS?

Practicing the movements slowly provides better control of body movement, clears of mind, and enhances concentration and relaxation.

IS IT TRUE THAT THE SLOWER ONE PRACTICES THE SOLO FORM THE BETTER?

Although the characteristic of tai chi chuan is to practice the solo form slowly, tai chi chuan has its own standard and one should practices according to that standard. Generally, it is slower for the beginner because one does not fully understand the form at that point. An experienced practitioner should practice the form more quickly because his body has adjusted to the movements.

The benefit of practicing the form more quickly will lead one to better mobility, quickness of movement, and ease of releasing power. Aside from being easier to learn, the benefits of practicing the form slowly will give one better coordination, concentration, balance, and body control.

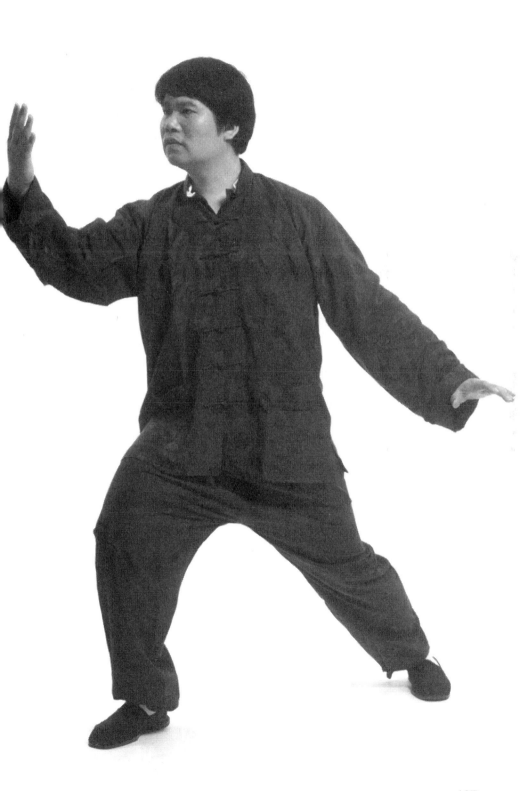

HOW SHOULD ONE BEGIN THEIR TAI CHI CHUAN PRACTICE?

First, you much seek out a well-trained and knowledgeable tai chi chuan instructor; not necessarily a "famous" instructor. Second, learn all of the postures, beginning with one posture at a time. Learn how the hands and feet move in each posture and how they coordinate with the body's weight. Third, after you have learned all of the postures, begin to refine them. Work on making the postures smooth, rounded, well-balanced, and coordinate them with the three human treasures: mind, power, and spirit. After you have completed this third level, you are considered as having achieved the beginning stages of tai chi chuan training.

WHY I AM NOT ABLE TO REMEMBER THE SOLO FORM POSTURES?

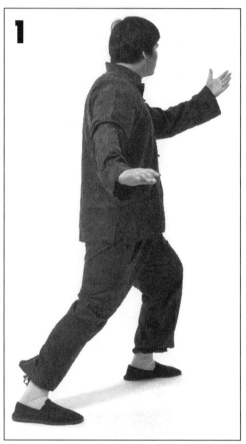

If you are having trouble remembering the sequence of postures, you are not alone. This happens to everyone at some time. The best method of remembering the postures is frequent practice and learning one posture at a time. Breakdown the movement into how the hands and feet move and how the body weight controls balance before moving on to another posture. In this way, you will truly understand every posture and will then not forget them as a whole.

WHAT ARE SOME OF THE FUNDAMENTALS OF THE STANCES IN TAI CHI CHUAN?

There are four major fundamentals to the stances in tai chi chuan that one needs to understand in order to improve their tai chi chuan training. Knowledge of these fundamentals is beneficial for both the beginners and experienced tai chi chuan practitioner.

1. The body weight is on the forward foot with the knee bent.

2. The body weight is on the backward foot with the knee bent.

3. The body weight is on both feet with the knees bent.

4. Standing on one leg.

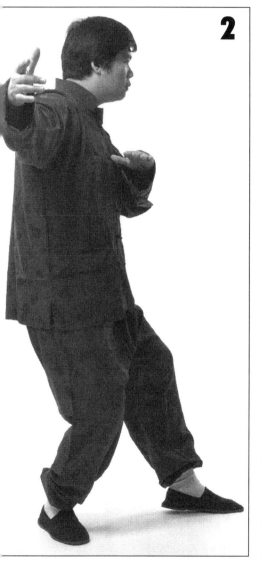
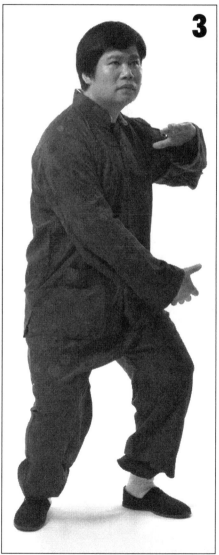

IS THE STUDY OF TAI CHI CHUAN ONLY FOR OLD PEOPLE?

Originally, tai chi chuan was famous as a martial art, and was not for old, sick, or weak people. However, as a result of its characteristics (i.e., slow, relax, concentrate, balance, and lightness), tai chi chuan became known for its value as a preventive therapy. For that, many older people practice it in the early mornings in parks, as is commonly seen in China. This gives people the impression that tai chi chuan is only for old people. However, as a result of its flexibility in practice, tai chi chuan can be of benefit for the old, sick, and weak as well as for young and strong people.

The martial art value of tai chi chuan requires that one has strong legs, good body condition, unity of mind, energy, and spirit. To achieve these requirements, one must engage in the complex and difficult training of tai chi chuan.

WHAT SHOULD THE BEGINNER CONCENTRATE ON?

Following is a list of the major things that one must pay attention to at all times, especially when first learning the solo form.

• **Correct posture: One must master the body, hands, and standing postures.**

• **Circular motion: One must keep in mind that there is circular motion in every movement of tai chi chuan.**

• **Lightness: One must be light in every movement, especially stepping of the feet, shifting of the body weight, and pushing of the hands forward.**

• **Slowness: One must be slow in all movements in order to have control, coordination, balance, and relaxation.**

• **Even: One must be sure to execute all movements at the same speed and keep their knees bent as the same height at all times.**

• **Balance: One must move the hands evenly throughout the form. In addition, the body weight must be supported on one foot before stepping with the other foot.**

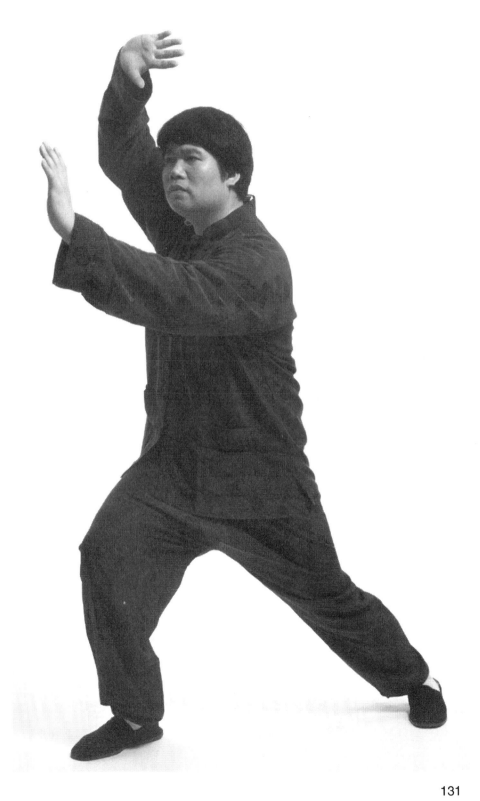

IS IT TRUE THAT IT IS BETTER TO KNOW MORE SOLO FORMS?

In the Yang style tai chi chuan system, there are the popular tai chi chuan and the cheung chuan forms. While similar, tai chi chuan emphasizes slowness in the form while cheung chuan emphasizes quickness in the form. If anyone is able to perfect these two forms, there is no need to learn the third form. These two forms contain enough training to perfect one as a human being and as a warrior.

WHEN DOES ONE DEVELOP A DEEP INTEREST
IN TAI CHI CHUAN?

At the beginning stages of training one does not tend to have much interest in the movements because they are difficult to remember. Interest will begin as soon as the beginner is able to master more movements, perhaps after six months of dedicated training.

WHAT IS THE BODY'S REQUIREMENT
IN PRACTICING TAI CHI CHUAN?

The main objective from the body in practicing tai chi chuan is to be held erect at all times. When this happens, the chest is sunk inward and the back is raised. The weight is sunk down to the bottom of the feet and the eyes look forward, the head suspended from above to lift the spirit.

HOW DO YOU DETERMINE IF A POSTURE IS CORRECT?

Outwardly, a posture is correct when it looks natural and comfortable. Inwardly, a posture is correct when one feels the energy coming from the feet to the hands. In order to have a correct posture, one should begin with the outward appearance. Following is a check list for this appearance:

- **Lower the elbows and relax the shoulders**

- **Bend the knees to line up with the toes**

- **Do not over extend the hands**

- **Keep your head upright and your eyes looking straight forward**

WHAT DOES IT MEAN TO USE THE MIND AND
NOT PHYSICAL POWER?

This means that when one practices a particular movement, one must pay attention to the detail of the hand and foot movement. One must understand the movement's usage and express this understanding outwardly without using physical power.

HOW DOES ONE ACHIEVE BALANCE IN TAI CHI CHUAN POSTURES AND MOVEMENTS?

In order to develop balance during practice, one must spend time strengthening the legs. A balanced stance begins with strong legs with which to root, wherein the toes act like nails anchored to the ground. Afterwards, one must understand the notion of being empty and full in movement by knowing when to use the hips to rotate the body and change weight when stepping.

WHY DO THE LEGS HURT WHEN ONE FIRST BEGINS TO STUDY TAI CHI?

When one practices tai chi chuan the knees are always bent, the movements executed slowly, and the body's weight supported by one leg at a time. These requirements put greater stress on the legs, thus making them painful for a time. However, after one has practiced for a period of time, leg strength will build and one will not have this problem again as the legs are stronger and thus able to support the body's weight. With this comes a better understand of the concept of full and empty.

WHAT DOES IT MEAN TO CALM THE MIND?

This means that there shall be no second thoughts in the mind when you are practicing tai chi chuan. The only things one needs to think about during practice is the correct movements of the hands and feet, thus allowing your brain a chance to rest and refresh itself. Therefore, people generally feel better after tai chi chuan practice.

WHAT DOES IT MEAN TO SUSPEND THE HEAD FROM ABOVE?

Originally, this was a story told about a scholar who hit his head on a table when he fell asleep while studying. In order to overcome this, he tied his hair to the rope which was suspended from the ceiling. Whenever his head fell forward, the rope would hold his head up and he would awaken to continue his study. In terms of tai chi chuan practice, suspend the head from above means that one must hold the head upright, keep the eyes looking forward, and hold the neck straight.

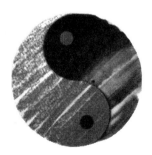

WHAT DOES IT TO MEAN RELAX?

In tai chi chuan, to relax does not mean to let go. In Chinese, this is referred to as *jou,* and is the combination of loose, relaxation, and hardness. In tai chi chuan practice, relaxation begins with sinking the shoulders and elbows, loosening all of the joins in the body. After years of practice, one will achieve the necessary relaxation. Yang Cheng Fu described this type of relaxation as "iron wrapped in cotton."

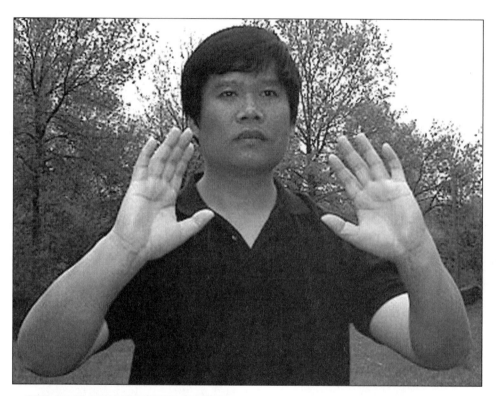

WHAT IS MEANT BY FLOWING?

In tai chi chuan practice, flowing refers to there being no breakage in any movement, meaning that all movements should be continuous from one posture to the next without a pause in between.

WHAT DOES IT MEAN TO SINK THE CHI DOWN TO THE DAN TIEN?

In order to practice this correctly, one should begin with the correct posture and breath with the diaphragm. If one's *chi* is successfully sinks down to the *dan tien* the lower abdomen will feel full, one's stance will be stronger, and their body more energetic.

WHAT IS MEANT BY NATURAL BREATHING?

Natural breathing is achieved when, on inhalation, the lower abdomen expands, and, on exhalation, the lower abdomen contracts.

WHAT IS MEANT BY DEEP BREATHING?

Deep breathing is when, upon inhalation, the diaphragm pushes downward and the lower abdomen extends outward. In turn, upon exhalation, the diaphragm contracts and the lower abdomen moves inward.

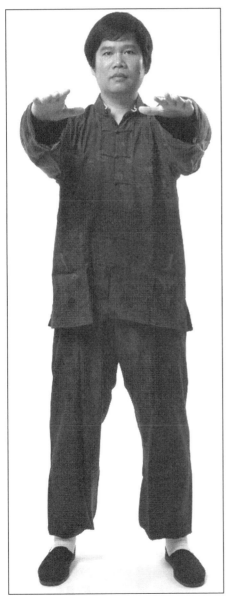 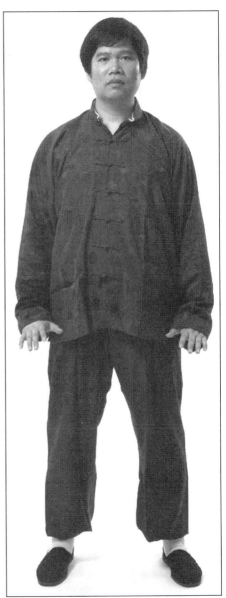

HOW DOES ONE COME TO UNDERSTAND OPEN AND CLOSE?

There are open and close movements everywhere in tai chi chuan. Open is the beginning of movement and close is the completion of a movement.

More specifically, open is the beginning of when the mind leads the *chi* to circulate throughout the body with the help of the physical movement. Therefore, it is said that when one practices the open movement, the entire body shall be open so that the *chi* will circulate through it. Close is the end of this *chi* circulation, wherein the energy returns back to the *dan tien*. Therefore, it is said that when a movement closes, the entire body is closed such that the *chi* can return back to the *dan tien*.

IS IT TRUE THAT A LARGE STANCE INHIBITS MOBILITY?

Yes, this is true. However, at the beginning one must have a large stance in order to facilitate proper balance and hip movement. A narrow stance in the beginning will provide the beginner with a narrow range of waist movement and perhaps develop bad habits later on.

IS IT TRUE THAT ONE SHOULD NOT MAKE A STANCE TOO LOW?

Generally, a lower stance is more stable and better for neutralizing techniques. High stances are not as stable but are better for mobility. Therefore, people practice with low stances and apply the techniques from high stances. Either way, a correct stance is formed when one leg is bent with its knee aligned with the toes while the second leg is kept straight.

SHOULD THE MOUTH BE OPEN OR CLOSED DURING TAI CHI CHUAN MOVEMENTS?

Tai chi chuan is an art of seeking stillness in movement. If the mouth is kept open to receive air, it will dry up rather quickly. Therefore, the mouth should be kept closed, with the tongue touching the roof to stimulate the production of more saliva. This is good for the digestive system and keeps the mouth moist.

HOW SHOULD THE HANDS BE FORMED IN TAI CHI CHUAN?

Relax the hands, with the fingers neither too close together nor too stiff. If the fingers curl or are stiff the *chi* will not be able to circulate there. When extended, the hands should not pass the knee in an effort to keep one from leaning too far forward.

WHY IS THIS ART CALLED TAI CHI CHUAN?

Tai chi chuan is a physical movement exercise based on the philosophy of tai chi or *yin/yang*. As such, tai chi chuan seeks out circular motion everywhere and each of the art's movements is composed of the *yin/yang* motion.

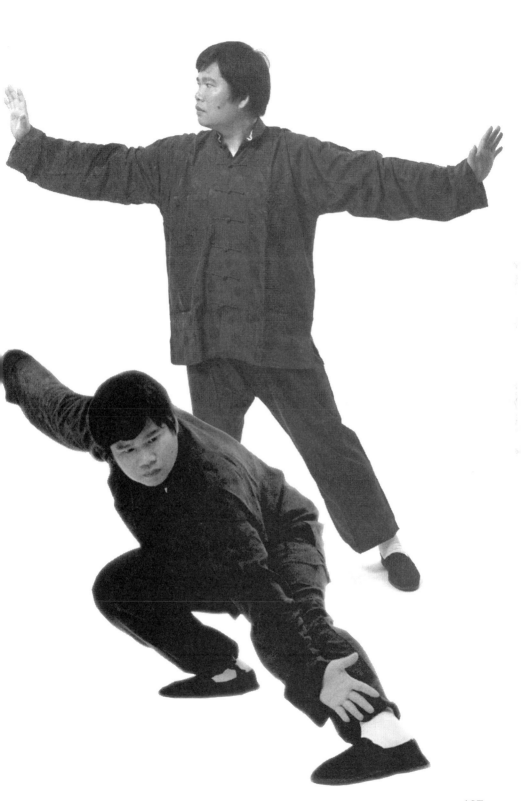

HOW DOES ONE MAINTAIN BALANCE IN TAI CHI CHUAN?

It is common among beginners of tai chi chuan to feel off-balance at times when holding certain postures. To begin with, one must recognize that during practice one is constantly shifting the body weight from one supporting leg to the other. In other words, if the left foot is solid, the entire body weight is on the left foot and the entire body depends on this foot for balance. Since all of the weight is supported on one foot in tai chi chuan, to maximize this support, the sole of the foot should be planted flat on the ground. In addition, the body must be held upright. If the body leans to either side, balance will be disrupted.

HOW CAN ONE IMPROVE THEIR TAI CHI CHUAN SKILLS?

To become good in tai chi chuan, one must follow the rules at all times, practicing all of the movements naturally and comfortably. If this is not done, then tai chi chuan will be of no benefit to the body.

In time, everything will come naturally. After one has learned the movements, one should begin to study and understand some of the concepts that underlie this art.

To become skillful in tai chi chuan, there is but one word: practice. It is said that after one practices the solo form thousands of times, its principles will begin to appear. Following is a list of the four things one needs to follow in order to become good at tai chi chuan:

• **More thinking: Use the head to find out why the movements move the way they do.**

• **Ask more questions: Aske all the question you may have.**

• **See more: spend more time observing how other people practice and take what is good.**

• **Practice more: The true way to learn is by actually practicing and not just talking about practicing.**

AFTERWORD

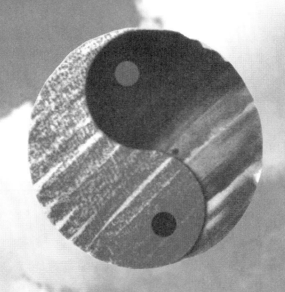

AFTERWORD

Ever since I first heard the comment that Grandmaster Yeung Sau Chung's book, *Practical Use of Tai Chi Chuan: Its Applications and Variations,* was great for people who have several years of tai chi chuan experience, but is untouchable for beginning students, the idea of publishing a book for beginners set in. I set my goal then to focus my teachings to prepare, lead, and guide practitioners to climb this tai chi chuan summit.

My friend and student, Rene Navarro, told me in one of the Friday evening classes that he was going to bring one of his friends from the book publication industry to visit out tai chi chuan school the following week. I asked Rene who his friend worked for, and Rene said that he did not know and had not actually met this new friend in person yet, but was told from a second friend that this friend just published a best selling book on Filipino martial arts. I was patiently awaiting his arrival. However, Rene told me the following week that his friend's visiting schedule canceled because he was tied up with work.

I met my publisher, Mr. Mark Wiley, in one of the Friday evening classes in 1997. That night, Rene offered my father and I a ride home with Mark sitting next to me in Rene's car. On our way home, Rene and Mark expressed their interest in the topic of beginner's books on tai chi and qigong, and would like to publish some in the future. I mentioned to Mark about Mr. Ou Wen Wei's qigong book and also my tai chi chuan book, which were for beginning students. Later, I asked Rene to pass my tai chi chuan and Mr. Ou's qigong manuscript on to Mark. Several weeks later I heard from Rene that Mark was interested in publishing both books.

I saw Mark several times at the school when he stopped by to gather photographs for Grandmaster Yeung's articles for his magazine *Martial Arts Illustrated.* Mark confirmed that he would indeed publish both books. I was thrilled and excited to know that my dream of publishing my book was becoming a reality.

Part of the original manuscript of this book was from a marketing class project I finished in college in the early 1980s. I recalled the professor told me that besides the typical marketing data and strategy analysis, it would be a better marketing project if I provided more background information about this unknown art, such as history, philosophy, and why so many people were doing it in China.

Since tai chi chuan is a novel art in this country, I was able to actually follow my marketing project's guidelines to make my contribution to popularize tai chi chuan. In the past several years, I published several articles in *Tai Chi* and *Inside Kung-Fu* magazines and I was invited to conduct workshops in

Vancouver, Canada in 1984. I also started to offer tai chi chuan classes at the Brookline Adult, Community, and Education Program, conducted workshops in France, The Czech Republic, and England, and began a cable television program teaching tai chi chuan on Brookline Access TV.

Publishing this book affirms my contribution to popularize this wonderful art of tai chi chuan in the United States. Over the years, people have doubted the accomplishments of the Yang style tai chi chuan practitioners. They said that it is impossible for a human being to achieve such skill and power. What these people do not know is how much work each practitioner has invested in his training. In the future, I will continue to publish work relating to this subject so that people will better comprehend the rich, informative, and guarded art of Yang style tai chi chuan.

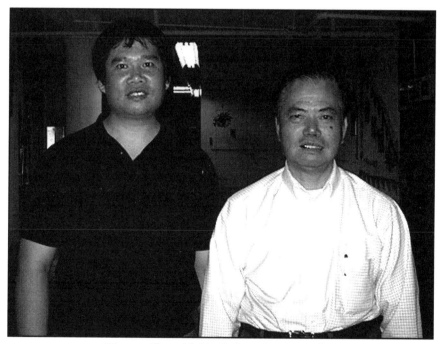

Vincent Chu with his Father, Gin Soon Chu.

THE GIN SOON TAI CHI CHUAN FEDERATION

The Gin Soon Tai Chi Club was founded in 1969 with permission from Grandmaster Yeung Sau Cheung to propagate the Yang style tai chi in North America. It is the oldest school teaching tai chi chuan in the Greater Boston Area today.

Although there are may schools of tai chi chuan in the United States, the Gin Soon Tai Chi Club is different from others because its founder, Master Gin Soon Chu, is a disciple who studied with and was authorized to teach by Grandmaster Yeung (Yang) Sau-Chung, firstborn and heir of the legendary Yang Cheng-fu. Master Chu received a deep and well-rounded training, first from Master Lai Hok Soon and then Grandmaster Yeung Sau-Cheung, a training that covered all aspects of classical Yang family tai chi chuan.

The school has reached many students from around the world with its traditional approach to training, characterized by personal individualized attention, emphasis on correct form, personal development, integration of body, *chi*, and intent, repetition, mutual respect, and hard work.

Over the years, many students have graduated from the school and became instructors themselves. In 1995, Gin Soon Tai Chi Federation was established to better serve our members who come from different countries.

We are receptive to teaching workshops, seminars, private or group classes at the headquarters and abroad. All the instructions are taught by Master Gin Soon Chu and his sons Vincent and Gordon Chu.

If you would like more information about Yang style tai chi chuan or the Gin Soon Tai Chi Chuan Federation, please feel free to contact us at:

Gin Soon Tai Chi Chuan Federation
33 Harrison Ave., 2nd Floor
Boston, MA 02111
(617) 542–4442
http://www.geocities.com/rodeodrive/4687

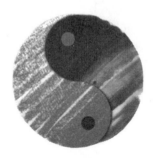

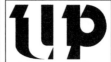

Multi-Media/Unique Publications
BOOK LIST

Action Kubotan Keychain: An Aid in Self-defense • Kubota, Takayuki • 1100
Advanced Balisong Manual, The • Imada, Jeff • 5192
Advanced Iron Palm • Gray, Brian • 416
Aikido: Traditional and New Tomiki • Higashi, Nobuyoshi • 319
American Freestyle Karate • Anderson, Dan • 303
Art of Stretching and Kicking, The • Lew, James • 206
Balisong Manual, The • Imada, Jeff • 5191
Beyond Kicking • Frenette, Jean • 421
Bruce Lee's One and Three Inch Power Punch • Demile, James • 502
Bruce Lee: The Biography • Clouse, Robert • 144
Bruce Lee: The Untold Story • Editors of Inside Kung-Fu • 401
Chi Kung: Taoist Secrets of Fitness & Longevity • Yu, Wen-Mei • 240
Chinese Healing Arts • Berk, William • 222
Choy Li Fut • Wong, Doc-Fai • 217
Complete Black Belt Hyung W.T.F., The • Cho, Hee Il • 584
Complete Guide to Kung-Fu Fighting Styles, The • Hallander, Jane • 221
Complete Iron Palm • Gray, Brian • 415
Complete Martial Artist Vol. 1, The • Cho, Hee Il • 5101
Complete Martial Artist Vol. 2, The • Cho, Hee Il • 5102
Complete Master's Jumping Kick, The • Cho, Hee Il • 581
Complete Master's Kick, The • Cho, Hee Il • 580
Complete One and Three Step Sparring, The • Cho, Hee Il • 582
Complete Tae Geuk Hyung W.T.F., The • Cho, Hee Il • 583
Complete Tae Kwon Do Hyung Vol. 1, The • Cho, Hee Il • 530
Complete Tae Kwon Do Hyung Vol. 2, The • Cho, Hee Il • 531
Complete Tae Kwon Do Hyung Vol. 3, The • Cho, Hee Il • 532
Deadly Karate Blows • Adams, Brian • 312
Deceptive Hands of Wing Chun, The • Wong, Douglas • 201
Dynamic Strength • Wong, Harry • 209
Dynamic Stretching and Kicking • Wallace, Bill • 405
Effective Techniques of Unarmed Combat • Hui, Mizhou • 130
Effortless Combat Throws • Cartmell, Tim • 261
Enter The Dragon Deluxe Collector's Set (25% max. discount) • Little, John • EDSP2
Essence of Aikido, The • Sosa, Bill • 320
Fatal Flute and Stick Form • Chan, Poi • 215
Fighting Weapons of Korean Martial Arts, The • Suh, In Hyuk • 355
Fundamentals of Pa Kua Chang, Vol. 1 • Nam, Park Bok • 245
Fundamentals of Pa Kua Chang, Vol. 2 • Nam, Park Bok • 246
Gene LeBell's Grappling World • LeBell, Gene • 593
Hapkido: The Integrated Fighting Art • Spear, Robert • 360
Hsing-I • McNeil, James • 225
Internal Secrets of Tai Chi Chuan • Wong, Doc-Fai • 250
Jackie Chan: The Best of Inside Kung-Fu • Little, John R. and Wong, Curtis F. • 599
Jean Frenette's Complete Guide to Stretching • Frenette, Jean • 420
Jeet Kune Do: Entering to Trapping to Grappling • Hartsell, Larry • 403

Multi-Media/Unique Publications
BOOK LIST

Jeet Kune Do: Its Concepts and Philosophies • Vunak, Paul • 410

Jeet Kune Do Kickboxing • Kent, Chris • 526

Jeet Kune Do Vol. 2: Counterattack, Grappling & Reversals • Hartsell, Larry • 404

Jeet Kune Do Unlimited • Richardson, Burton • 440

Jo: The Japanese Short Staff • Zier, Don • 310

Jun Fan Jeet Kune Do: The Textbook • Kent, Chris • 528

Kata and Kumite for Karate • Thompson, Chris • 558

Kendo: The Way and Sport of the Sword • Finn, Michael • 562

Kenjustu: The Art of Japanese Swordsmanship • Daniel, Charles • 323

Kokushi-ryu Jujutsu • Higashi, Nobuyoshi • 322

Koryu Aikido • Higashi, Nobuyoshi • 321

Kung-Fu: History, Philosophy, and Techniques • Chow, David • 103

Kung-Fu: The Endless Journey • Wong, Douglas • 230

Kung-Fu: The Way of Life • Wong, Douglas • 202

Making of Enter the Dragon, The • Clouse, Robert • 145

Man of Contrasts • Cho, Hee Il • 508

Martial Arts Around the World • Soet, John • 140

Ninjutsu History and Tradition • Hatsumi, Masaaki • 105

Northern Sil Lum #7, Moi Fah • Lam, Kwong Wing • 213

Nunchaku: The Complete Guide • Shiroma, Jiro • $12.95

Pangu Mystical Qigong • Wei, Ou Wen • 242

Practical Chin Na • Yuan, Zhao Da • 260

Science of Martial Arts Training, The • Staley, Charles I. • 445

Searching for the Way • Sutton, Nigel • 180

Secret History of the Sword, The • Amberger, J. Christoph • 150

Shaolin Chin Na • Yang, Jwing-Ming • 207

Shaolin Fighting Theories and Concepts • Wong, Douglas • 205

Shaolin Five Animals Kung-Fu • Wong, Doc-Fai • 218

Shaolin Long Fist Kung-Fu • Yang, Jwing-Ming • 208

Study of Form Mind Boxing • Tang, Sun Lu • 235

Tai Chi for Two: The Practice of Push Hands • Crompton, Paul • 568

Tai Chi Sensing Hands • Olson, Stuart A. • 287

Tai Chi Thirteen Sword: A Sword Master's Manual • Olson, Stuart A. • 285

Tai Chi Training in China: Masters, Teachers & Coaches • Thomas, Howard • 567

Taijutsu: Ninja Art of Unarmed Combat • Daniel, Charles • 125

Tang Soo Do: The Ultimate Guide to the Korean Martial Art • Lee, Kang Uk • 585

Traditional Ninja Weapons • Daniel, Charles • 108

Training and Fighting Skills • Urquidez, Benny • 402

Tomiki Aikido: Randori & Koryu No Kata • Loi, Lee Ah • 551

Total Quality Martial Arts • Hess, Christopher D. • 447

Ultimate Kick, The • Wallace, Bill • 406

Warrior Walking • Holzer, Josh • 155

Warrior Within: The Mental Approach of a Champion • Brewerton, Kevin • 450

Wing Chun Bil Jee • Cheung, William • 214

Wu Style of Tai Chi Chuan, The • Lee, Tinn Chan • 211

Xing Yi Nei Gong • Miller, Dan • 226

Yang Style Tai Chi Chuan • Yang, Jwing-Ming • 210

Yuen Kay-San Wing Chun Kuen • Ritchie, Rene • 275-1